Thanks for the Love!

PRAISE FOR THE VegNews GUIDE TO BEING A FABULOUS VEGAN

"*The VegNews Guide to Being a Fabulous Vegan* provides a refreshing perspective on how to get animal products out of your diet and embrace a life that is in line with your values. If you're curious about veganism, start right here." —**JOAQUIN PHOENIX,** Academy Award, Grammy, and Golden Globe Winner

"From the delicious and easy recipes to longtime VegNews editor Jasmin Singer's insightful, fun, and informative commentary, every part of *The VegNews Guide to Being a Fabulous Vegan* is truly fabulous. I only wish I had this book when I started eating plant-based! Whether you're ready to make a change in your life or just leaning into this wonderful, conscientious, ethical, and delicious diet, *The VegNews Guide to Being a Fabulous Vegan* is a must-read." —**DAISY FUENTES**, TV host and entrepreneur

"Never did I think I would find a book that held so many things I care and love about so perfectly in one place. *The VegNews Guide to Being a Fabulous Vegan* eases you in, helping you to not only make a healthier dietary decision for yourself but also educating you on why veganism is important as a movement. Chockfull of every single delicious alternative you can think of, as well as mouthwatering photos, this book is my new vegan bible!" —**MENA SUVARI**, actor

"As a dedicated vegan and parent to vegan children, VegNews has long been a staple in my life. Jasmin Singer has taken the approachable, fun, delicious, and meaningful experience that is VegNews and folded it into this incredible book—which is the only book you need to own if you are vegan or even just vegan-curious. VegNews and Singer have created such a glorious vegan book, and I can't wait to send this to everyone (vegan and non-vegan) I know." —**MAYIM BIALIK**, actor and bestselling author

"I've been an admirer of both VegNews and Singer's incredible vegan advocacy for years, and I am thrilled and grateful they have distilled their substantial knowledge and insights about the vegan lifestyle into a book that will undoubtedly help you with every aspect of plant-based living. From making sure your mascara wasn't tested on bunnies to figuring out what to eat for breakfast to getting a grasp on the role animal agriculture has on the environment (and what you can do about it), *The VegNews Guide to Being a Fabulous Vegan* is the book I'll be giving to new and seasoned vegan friends alike!" —**EVANNA LYNCH**, actor

"For the sake of the environment alone, more than ever, shifting to a vegan diet is crucial. If there is not a planet healthy enough for all living beings to healthfully inhabit, not one other issue great or small—from animal rights to civil rights to voting in elections—will matter. *The VegNews Guide to Being a Fabulous Vegan* is essential in helping make the surprisingly easy and delectable switch to plant-based."

—**TIG NOTARO**, comedian and Grammy Award winner

"*The VegNews Guide to Being a Fabulous Vegan* is sassy, smart, and full of thousands of tips for ditching animal products, and delivered in a digestible way that literally anyone can implement. As you read this book, Jasmin Singer will become your best friend—the kind that knows more than you, but invites you in rather than pushes you out. Get ready to have your mind blown. After reading *The VegNews Guide to Being a Fabulous Vegan*, your life will never be the same."

—**DANIELLA MONET**, actress and influencer

"Veganism has moved from fringe to mainstream, and *The VegNews Guide to Being a Fabulous Vegan* is there for anyone who is ready to make a choice that honors their values of not hurting animals, protecting the planet, and embracing the best food on the planet. Everything about this book is—as promised—totally fabulous, and Jasmin Singer is both deeply thoughtful and totally hilarious in her writing."

—**JANE VELEZ-MITCHELL**, *New York Times* bestselling author and TV host

THE VegNews GUIDE TO BEING A
FABULOUS VEGAN

LOOK GOOD, FEEL GOOD
& DO GOOD IN 30 DAYS

JASMIN SINGER & VegNews MAGAZINE

Go
hachette
BOOKS
NEW YORK

Hachette Go, an imprint of Hachette Books
Hachette Book Group
1290 Avenue of the Americas
New York, NY 10104
HachetteGo.com
Facebook.com/HachetteGo
Instagram.com/HachetteGo

First Edition: December 2020
Hachette Books is a division of Hachette Book Group, Inc.
The Hachette Go and Hachette Books name and logos are trademarks of Hachette Book Group, Inc.
The publisher is not responsible for websites (or their content) that are not owned by the publisher.

Print book interior design by Tabitha Lahr.

Library of Congress Cataloging-in-Publication Data

Names: Singer, Jasmin, author.
Title: The VegNews guide to being a fabulous vegan: look good, feel good,
   & do good in 30 days / Jasmin Singer & VegNews magazine.
Other titles: Veg News guide to being a fabulous vegan | VegNews Magazine.

Description: First edition. | New York, NY: Hachette Books, 2020. |
   Includes bibliographical references and index.
Identifiers: LCCN 2020014609 | ISBN 9780306846182 (paperback) | ISBN
   9780306846175 (ebook)
Subjects: LCSH: Vegan cooking. | Cooking (Natural foods) | International
   cooking. | LCGFT: Cookbooks.
Classification: LCC TX837 .S524 2020 | DDC 641.5/6362—dc23
LC record available at https://lccn.loc.gov/2020014609
ISBNs: 978-0-306-84618-2 (paperback); 978-0-306-84617-5 (ebook)

Printed in China

IM

10 9 8 7 6 5 4 3 2 1

CONTENTS

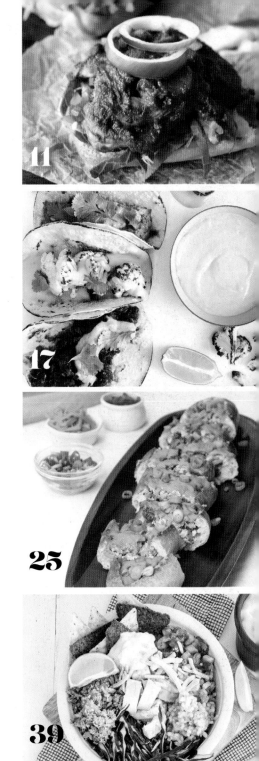

11

17

25

39

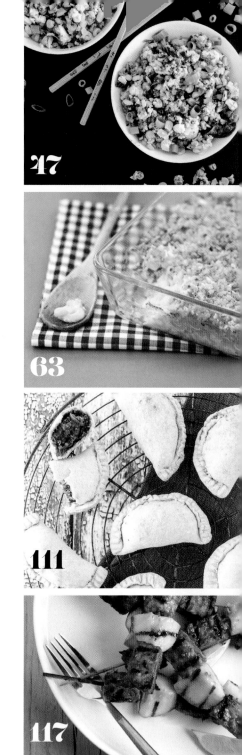

117

63

111

117

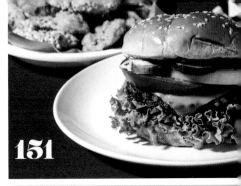

151

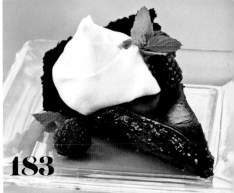

183

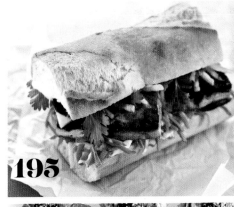

195

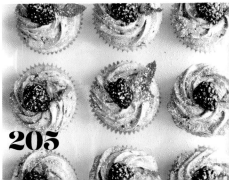

205

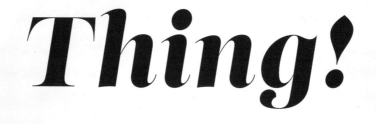

Caring . . . It's a Thing!

Day 1

*The best thing for you is the best thing for the planet, the best thing for the people of the world, and the best thing for the animals. And the greatest part of it all? It's so damn **delicious**.*

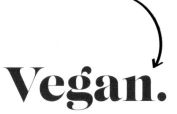

Vegan.

There are few other words in the English language that immediately bring up such a knee-jerk reaction among pretty much everyone. Of course, you've got your stereotypes (vegans are weak, they're angry, they're hippies, they're annoying, they're probably right); your immediate defenses ("If I go vegan, I'd miss my mom's amazing Christmas pot roast, and I won't be able to put creamer in my coffee"); and—admit it—your curiosity ("Veganism does seem to be the best way to lower my carbon footprint . . . Not to mention, I just saw some supercute new vegan shoes that I kind of want"). Anyone who has ever considered going entirely plant-based—whether or not they ever followed through—has struggled with the exact same questions, faced identical food-scarcity fears, and wondered whether it was healthy. Let's just start off right now by saying that you—as well as your skepticism and intrigue—are not alone.

The fact that you're even reading this is indication enough that this book is for you, because regardless of where you fall on the vegan-curious spectrum—from "My girlfriend gave me this book and told me I have to read it or she'll break up with me" to "Here! Take my leather belt! Where can I get a hemp replacement? I'm all in!"—leaning into plant-based living, whether you want to try it for a month or you're ready to go full-throttle, has something for everybody.

There's so much we can't control. Politics. Missed trains. Elevator music. What our ex says about us.

And yet there is so much we *can* control. How we react to missing that train. The song we rebelliously sing in our head when the elevator music is making us fall asleep. The choice to finally block our ex on social media.

What we eat. What we don't.

In today's tech-driven, fast-paced world, there is solace and order in the power that comes when we align our values with what we consume. It's something we *do* have control over. For most of us, pushing past our comfort zone long enough to ask ourselves the tough questions—whether our diet truly matches our vision for how we want to feel—results in an often indisputable shift toward eating plants.

Veganism. There's that word again . . . the one that bounces around our head when we stare at the late-night menu selections at the diner and momentarily question whether that hamburger is really the right choice. Won't it make us feel sluggish and heavy? Why does it seem so viscerally disgusting to so many of us? Or what about those of us for whom meat is extra tasty, a fact that secretly riddles us with guilt? Yet we order it anyway, because that's just what we do.

But it doesn't have to be. In fact, it can't be. Since the advent of factory farming in the 1950s, the animal agriculture industry has created a monstrosity of epic proportions that is entirely unsustainable any way you look at it—both for the planet and for our own bodies. Speaking of our glorious bodies, when it comes to feeling great so that we can perform as best as possible at the gym, the answer is simple: we have to start fueling ourselves with plants. And fear not, because veganism today is not your mother's vegetarianism of yesterday.

When you're talking about stepping up your fitness game, the easiest and most effective answer is to go vegan. Whether it's long-distance runners, weightlifters, baseball players, football players, or tennis players, so many of the people who are truly interested in optimizing their health—world-class athletes—are turning to vegan diets and experiencing incredible results. The evidence is piling up that plant-based eating is not only possible from a nutritional perspective, but it's the healthiest possible way to feed yourself.

In fact, plant-based diets can help prevent all sorts of diseases, from heart disease to type 2 diabetes, rheumatoid arthritis, stroke, obesity, and the myriad other chronic diseases plaguing America, including many forms of cancer. Plants are incredibly good for you and have all sorts of nutrients that are absolutely crucial for optimal health and fitness. As you'll see in these pages, plant-based food also tastes totally fantastic.

While most of us know that too much of these animal-derived foods are unhealthy, until recently, we didn't realize that we didn't need them at all, and that plants are truly where it's at when it comes to optimal health, the health of our planet, and our collective care of individual animals.

This book is going to break all of that down in really specific ways that will set you up for success. We will delve into common questions about things like protein (spoiler alert: vegans get plenty, and they get it from the same exact place as rhinos and elephants); things that everyone wonders but no one

A History Lesson

Dick Gregory (1932–2017) was a social justice pioneer, a civil rights movement hero, and a gifted comedian. He was also an outspoken vegan, often giving talks on the nutritional considerations, economic impacts, and cultural foundations of why Black Americans evolved to eat meat-heavy diets, and advocated for Black people to stop eating animals.

> *I had been a participant in all of the "major" and most of the "minor" civil rights demonstrations of the early sixties. Under the leadership of Dr. King, I became convinced that nonviolence meant opposition to killing in any form. I felt the commandment "Thou Shalt Not Kill" applied to human beings not only in their dealings with each other—war, lynching, assassination, murder, and the like—but in their practice of killing animals for food and sport. Animals and humans suffer and die alike. Violence causes the same pain, the same spilling of blood, the same stench of death, the same arrogant, cruel, and brutal taking of life.*

> **—DICK GREGORY**, from his memoir, *Callus on My Soul*

asks (another spoiler alert: yes, breast milk is vegan, and yes, vegans have better sex); and things that you didn't realize you need to know, but now you're so glad you do (no, you don't need to keep swallowing expensive, inhumane fish oil to get your omegas).

A really common concern people have when going vegan is the perceived permanence of the word. It can indeed sound really big and really serious, especially if the only vegans you know exist online. Let this book help you ease into veganism, taking it one day at a time so that you don't get overwhelmed by all the things you're worried about and then don't try at all. This book is not about perfection, and neither is veganism.

So, try it for thirty days in a row. Or not in a row. Make all of the mouthwatering recipes in these pages, or just read them as you snack on popcorn. Read a chapter every morning, or read this whole book in one weekend. Buy a copy for your skeptical dad so he can understand why you're doing this cockamamie thing, or get a copy for your newly vegan cousin—or give yourself the gift of keeping it all for you.

There are no rules for reading this book, and there are no rules for going vegan.

Wait, that's not true. There's one rule: don't eat or use animal products. That's what *vegan* means, and it's easier—and more interesting and fun and fashionable and delicious—than you think.

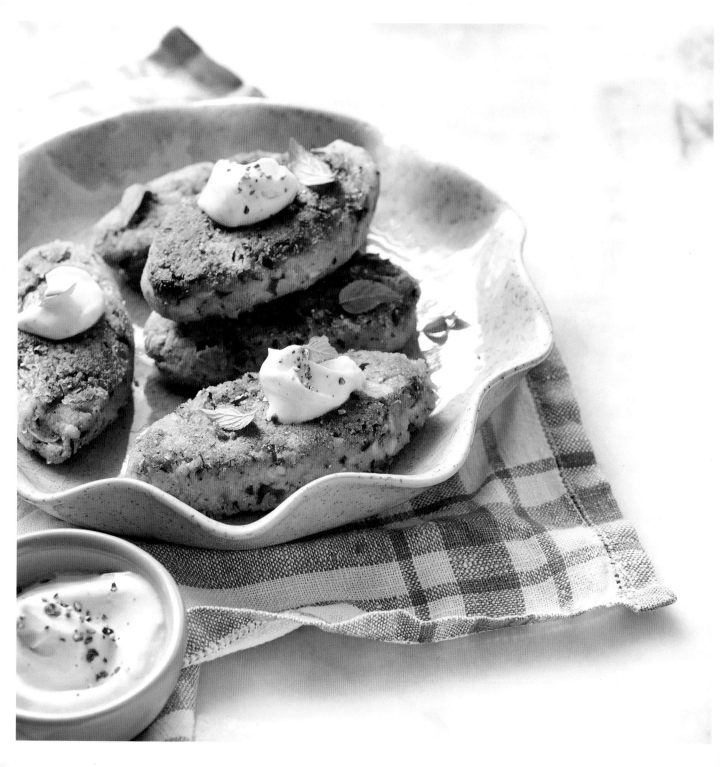

Black-Eyed Pea Croquettes with Creamy Rémoulade Sauce

Packed with protein, black-eyed peas are also believed to be good luck when eaten at the beginning of the year. But you'll certainly be feeling lucky with these crisp, light croquettes—drizzled in creamy French sauce—all year round.

Croquettes:

1   tablespoon plus 2 teaspoons safflower oil
½   medium-size onion, finely chopped
2   garlic cloves, finely chopped
1   small zucchini, finely chopped
½   red bell pepper, seeded and finely chopped
1   (15-ounce) can organic black-eyed peas, drained and rinsed
½   teaspoon seafood seasoning
½   teaspoon salt
¼   teaspoon freshly ground black pepper
2   tablespoons vegan Worcestershire sauce
2   tablespoons freshly squeezed lemon juice
1½ teaspoons pure maple syrup
½   cup finely ground yellow cornmeal
½   cup bread crumbs

Rémoulade sauce:

2   tablespoons vegan sour cream
3   tablespoons vegan mayonnaise
½   teaspoon hot sauce
1   teaspoon freshly squeezed lemon juice
Zest of ½ lemon
¾   teaspoon pure maple syrup
¼   teaspoon salt
¼   teaspoon freshly ground black pepper

1 **Prepare the croquettes:** In a sauté pan over medium heat, heat 2 teaspoons of oil. Add onion, garlic, zucchini, and bell pepper and cook for 3 to 5 minutes to soften. Transfer the mixture to a large bowl. Set aside.

2 In a food processor, combine black-eyed peas, seafood seasoning, salt, black pepper, Worcestershire sauce, lemon juice, maple syrup, cornmeal, and bread crumbs. Pulse until mixture is even and smooth. Transfer to a bowl and fold in vegetables.

3 In a large skillet over medium heat, heat remaining tablespoon of oil. With damp hands, form ¼ cup portions of croquette mixture into football shapes about ½ inch thick. Place in pan and cook for 3 to 5 minutes on each side, or until golden and warmed through.

4 **Prepare the rémoulade sauce:** Combine all sauce ingredients in a medium bowl and whisk together.

5 To serve, dollop each warm croquette with sauce.

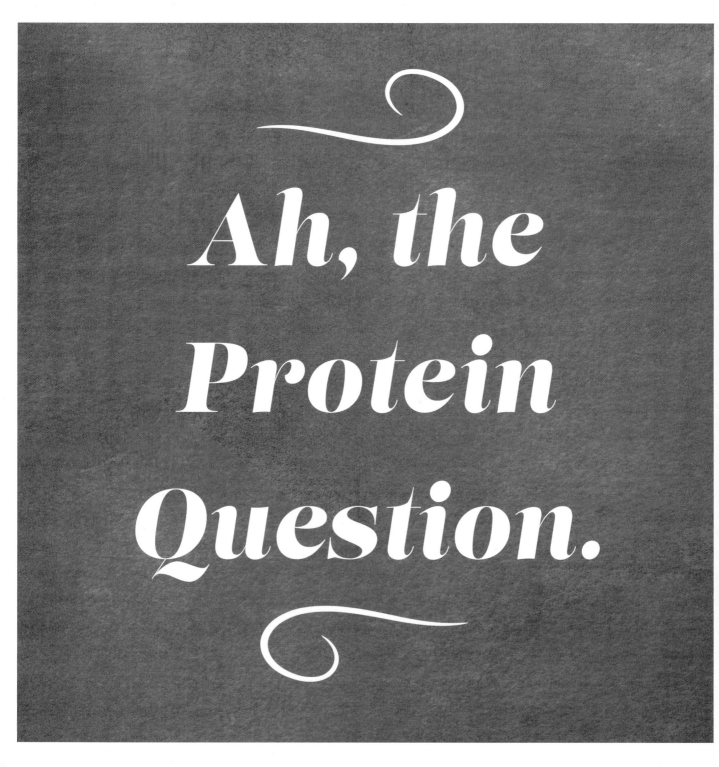

Day 2

*You'll get your protein from the same place as the elephants, giraffes, and moose: **nutrition-packed plants**.*

Look around.

Do Americans look like they have a protein deficit, or a deficit of anything? We are hardly a country full of people who are wilting away. The "protein question"—which vegans are very, very used to being asked—is almost always worthy of an eye roll, but the truth is, folks really, actually want to know. It has been drummed into our head that we need a lot more protein than we actually do, and that animal flesh is the best way to achieve that. Yet all of that is severely misguided. Slow your roll, because we can absolutely get more than sufficient protein on a vegan diet.

A whole lot of experts and medical professionals underline this point. The Academy of Nutrition and Dietetics—the United States' largest conglomerate of food and nutrition professionals (representing over 100,000 registered nutritionists and technicians)—has stated, "Plant protein can meet requirements when a variety of plant foods is consumed and

energy needs are met." There you have it. Feel free to move on to the next chapter now. (Just kidding. Keep reading this one first.)

And the myth that vegans don't get enough protein is just part of it; the other side of the story is that, in general, most people get way too much protein. Have you ever heard of *kwashiorkor*? Probably not. Kwashiorkor is protein malnutrition caused by famine, and—though extremely rare—is seen mostly in undeveloped countries; harrowing images of starving children with big bellies and skinny limbs might come to mind. The reason we don't see it in developed countries, such as the United States, is that it's very uncommon. Although there are instances in the United States where someone might have less-than-adequate protein (but not kwashiorkor) this is also extremely rare because there's protein in everything.

And we do mean everything. Vegans specifically get protein from healthy and robust foods, including lentils, beans, seeds, nuts, whole grains (such as quinoa and oats), fruit, vegetables (bok choy, kale), soy products (tofu, tempeh, edamame), and seitan (vegan meats).

If you dive into the protein question, you will find there are two other related questions: "What is a complete protein?" and "Do I need to combine foods to get a complete protein?" It takes twenty different amino acids to make protein; some of these are made from our bodies, while others—essential amino acids (EAA)—have to be provided by what we eat. To get enough EAA, we need to keep filling up with a variety of plant foods so that we can replenish our supply. The antiquated idea, popularized in the 1970s, that we need to combine foods to get a perfect protein—such as eating beans and rice together (but not individually)—has been wildly disproven. As long as we're eating a variety of plant-based foods, we will obtain all the complete protein we need. In fact, we will thrive. As long as we eat our beans.

If it calls to you to actually calculate how much protein you need, follow this rule: Adults should eat 0.36 grams a day for every pound of healthy body weight (if you're 150 pounds, that equals about 60 grams of protein per day). You really don't need to overthink this, though. If you're taking in enough calories and are eating mostly whole foods—again, that's vegetables, beans, fruit, and whole grains—you will get enough protein. Pinkie swear.

Another way of looking at it is to aim for three to four servings of legumes each day (one serving can look like ½ cup of cooked beans, tofu, or tempeh; 2 tablespoons of peanut butter; or ¼ cup of peanuts). Word to the wise: split peas or lentils are less gas-producing *and* higher in protein because they are nonbean legumes (you're welcome). One other thing to keep in mind is that as far as dairy-free milks go, soy milk and pea milk (yes, pea milk is a thing, and the brand Ripple makes it particularly well) have more protein than almond, rice, oat, and hemp.

Much like religion, our deeply ingrained mindsets around food often present themselves in our conversations and blindly dictate our meal choices. The idea that we don't get enough protein without meat is so completely absurd (do you actually know anyone who has ever suffered from protein deficiency?), and yet it's in many of our go-to belief systems. But why? The meat industrial complex and dairy lobby force-feed us this kind of messaging, starting when we are little kids and are told that milk "does a body good" and that meat and dairy are required for strength and optimal nutrition. There is big money behind these kinds of misperceptions, and these mega-companies are literally relying on our willful ignorance to eat it up. Our suggestion is to spit it out instead.

So, the next time a meat-eater asks you where you get your protein, you might want to respond by asking them where they get theirs. Then, you have full permission to rip this page out and hand it to them (whether you ask them to actually eat this page is totally up to you). Then, take them out for a bucket of seitan wings, your treat.

Packs a Punch

You want protein? We've got protein.

LENTILS	18 grams per 1 cup serving
EDAMAME	17 grams per 1 cup serving
SEITAN	16 grams per 2 ounce serving
TEMPEH	15 grams per ½ cup serving
TOFU	10 grams per ½ cup serving
HEMP SEEDS	10 grams per 3 tablespoon serving
GREEN PEAS	8 grams per 1 cup serving
PEANUT BUTTER	8 grams per 2 tablespoon serving
QUINOA	8 grams per 1 cup serving
SOY MILK	8 grams per 1 cup serving
BLACK BEANS	7.5 grams per ½ cup serving
CHICKPEAS	7.5 grams per 1 cup serving
PINTO BEANS	7 grams per ½ cup serving
WILD RICE	7 grams in 1 cup serving
STEEL-CUT OATS	5 grams per ¼ cup serving, dry
SPIRULINA	4 grams per 1 tablespoon serving
CHIA SEEDS	4 grams per 2 tablespoon serving
KALE	3 grams per 1 cup serving
BROCCOLI	2.4 grams per 1 cup serving

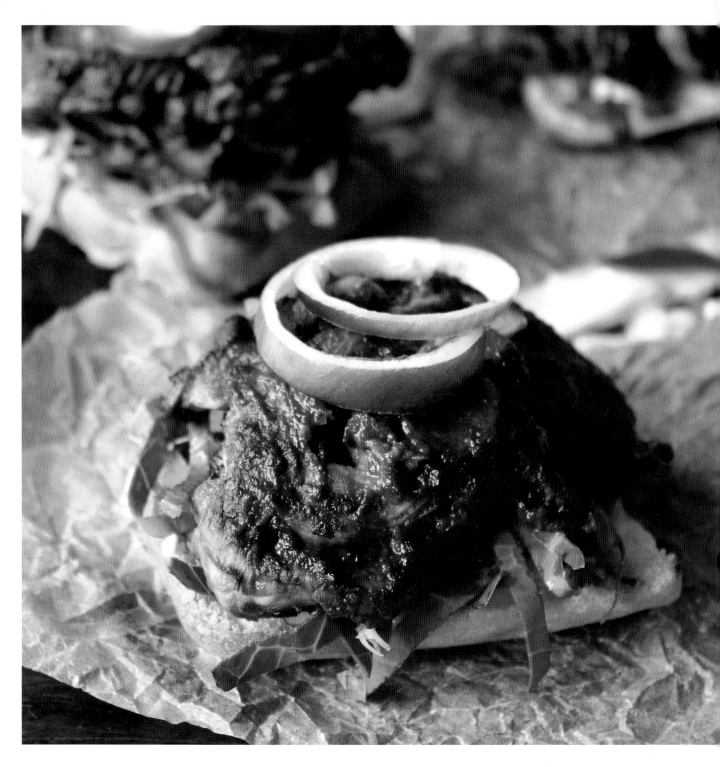

BBQ Oyster Mushroom Sliders

Marvelously meaty mushrooms are made even tastier with a quick sear and a basting of smoky-sweet barbecue sauce.

1	tablespoon grapeseed oil
8	ounces (4 cups) oyster mushrooms, cut into 3-inch pieces
¼	teaspoon salt
1	cup vegan barbecue sauce
4	small vegan ciabatta buns

1	cup thinly sliced collard greens
2	teaspoons olive oil
¼	cup vegan mayonnaise
½	medium-size red onion, thinly sliced

1 In a cast-iron skillet over medium-high heat, heat grapeseed oil. Place mushrooms, cut side down, in skillet and sprinkle with salt. Lower heat to medium-low.

2 Place another cast-iron skillet on top of mushrooms. Cook for 7 minutes, flip mushrooms, and continue to cook between both skillets for 5 more minutes, or until browned and tender.

3 Pour barbecue sauce over mushrooms and gently stir to coat. Continue to cook, uncovered, for 5 more minutes.

4 To assemble sliders, toast buns on each side. Massage collard greens with olive oil for 3 minutes, or until tender. Spread 1 tablespoon mayonnaise on each bun. Top bottom bun with collards, then add oyster mushrooms. Top with a few slices of red onion and top bun. Serve immediately.

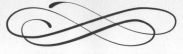

Not Just a Passing Trend!

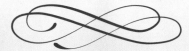

Day 3

*The practice of leaving animal products off your plate is older than time; it existed before Beyoncé, before Instagram, and **before your great-great-great grandparents were putting supper on the table.***

Boomerang.

Pet celebrities. Smoothie bowls. They are Instagram-worthy, shocking, and fleeting. Although some trends find their way back to the zeitgeist, whims pass for a reason. In diet-speak, we've seen everything from the watermelon diet to the carb-free diet, the carb-only diet to the eat-every-other-day diet. Low-fat, high-fat, low-carb, all-meat, keto, paleo, Atkins . . . you get the picture. Diets come and go, but veganism—a term coined in 1944 by British activist Donald Watson—is no passing thing.

In the last few years, veganism officially entered the mainstream. Research firm Global Data compiled a report that highlighted six key trends in the worldwide prepared foods industry, two of which—"go meat-free" and "ethical eating"—specifically centered on eliminating or reducing animal products. The keen interest in ditching animal products cannot be denied and is further proven by the fact that the number of Americans identifying as vegan has gone up by 600 percent in just three years. This explosive growth is influenced by a myriad of factors, including the environmental and health benefits of eliminating animal products, the ethics of leaving animals off our plates, and (for better or for worse) an onslaught of countless celebrities who are suddenly hashtagging things #vegan. Veganism is not just a trend, but a lifestyle choice that's dislodging itself from the margins and becoming the norm.

The surging popularity of veganism is far-reaching, with worldwide implications and manifestations. Around the globe, people are making the connection. Plant-based companies in Brazil are growing at a rate of 40 percent annually. In China, the vegan population has increased to more than fifty million. CNN recently posited that Germany is leading the way for a vegan revolution, pointing to the exponential growth of vegan products being released in the country faster than you can say *Ach du lieber Gott!* (a whopping one in ten of all new products there are entirely plant-based). In Canada, 53 percent of residents consume meat alternatives. Omnipork, a brand-new plant-based product that mimics the flavor, consistency, and versatility of ground pork, recently launched in Hong Kong at the Michelin-starred, Cantonese fine-dining restaurant Ming Court. In the United Kingdom, there are an estimated 3.5 million vegans. In the Middle East, Prince Khaled bin Alwaleed bin Talal of Saudi Arabia announced his plans to open at least ten vegan restaurants in an effort to boycott fast-food eateries, empower people to reach their optimal health, and combat the obesity epidemic that he says is a disaster plaguing the region.

And this craze is nothing new. Although it's been in the spotlight more and more—especially as enormous fast-food chains introduce vegan options (Burger King, Carl's Jr., and even KFC now offer vegan versions of traditional, animal-based menu items), plant-based eating is as old as food itself. Those who follow such religions as Buddhism, Jainism, and Seventh-Day Adventism pretty much wrote that book. Japanese Buddhist monks were practically donning vegan message-wear back in the sixth century when they created the cuisine known as *shojin ryori*, a type of vegetarian cooking focused around simple tastes and fresh foods. And Seventh-Day Adventists—veg for over 150 years—are known for their long life expectancy. By the time the term *vegan* was actually coined, eschewing animal products was old hat. And by the time Miley Cyrus

caught wind of the benefits of a vegan diet in 2014, animal studies had already been an official degree for students studying at New York University.

Veganism has deep roots in Africa, too. Precolonial Africans relied heavily on plants, making up the bulk of their diet. It was a mix of globalization and cultural appropriation that caused many African societies to revolve around meat. But prior to farming, Africans were hunters and gatherers, focusing their finds on vegetables, including tubers, bulbs, and edible flowers—with the occasional game. It wasn't until just five centuries ago, when slave-traders showed up, that larger-scale crops—such as animals used for food—were introduced, becoming a lucrative field and changing the shape of how Africans ate.

So, veganism is clearly no breeze-through novelty. Its roots have been planted for eons, and it is the only way forward. And whether the global shift to plant-based living is based on health (the United Nations has stated that a well-planned vegan diet can be optimal); athleticism (the rise in vegan athletes is exponential, as evidenced by the 2019 James Cameron–produced Sundance documentary *The Game Changers* highlighting multiple professional champion athletes from the NFL, NBA, and WWF); the environment (the carbon footprint of people who eat meat every day outweighs the footprint produced by vegans by 1.8 tons); or ethics (more than fifty billion land animals worldwide are raised and slaughtered for meat annually); all signs point to veganism as the sustainable and sound lifestyle choice. There is nothing fleeting about that.

Veganism Throughout Time

The roots of veganism go back further than you might think.

500 BCE—Greek philosopher and mathematician Pythagoras of Samos preaches compassion toward all sentient beings (as well as much ado about triangles)

1748—Famed utilitarian philosopher Jeremy Bentham is born. During his career, he teaches that animal suffering is equal to human suffering and considers the concept of human species superiority a form of racism

1850—Rev. Sylvester Graham, the inventor of graham crackers, founds the American Vegetarian Society

1942—Sir Paul McCartney—soon to be a ridiculously famous member of the Beatles—is born, and will go on to mainstream animal advocacy issues, such as fighting seal hunting

1944—British activist Donald Watson officially coins the term *vegan* and also founds the Vegan Society

1960—Jay Dinshah founds the American Vegan Society, based on Watson's work, effectively bringing veganism to the States

1987—Iconic electronic musician Moby goes vegan, then dedicates his life to animal advocacy—influencing millions of his fans to try plant-based on for size

1995—Coretta Scott King, activist and widow of Dr. Martin Luther King Jr., is convinced by her son Dexter to adopt a vegan diet

2010—Vegan ultra-endurance athlete Rich Roll completes the EPIC5 Challenge, finishing five Ironmans on the five islands of Hawaii in just over five consecutive days

2016—Ben & Jerry's launches its first four nondairy flavors in the United States

2017—*Orange Is the New Black* actress Ruby Rose fully commits to a vegan diet following an unpleasant memory of shark fin soup

2018—ESPN and *USA Today* reveal that fifteen Tennessee Titans have committed to Chef Charity Morgan's (wife of Titans linebacker Derrick Morgan) vegan meal plan

2019—Vegan meat brand Beyond Meat goes public, raising its IPO price from an initial $46 to a closing price of $65.75, making it the best-performing IPO on the market in nearly two decades

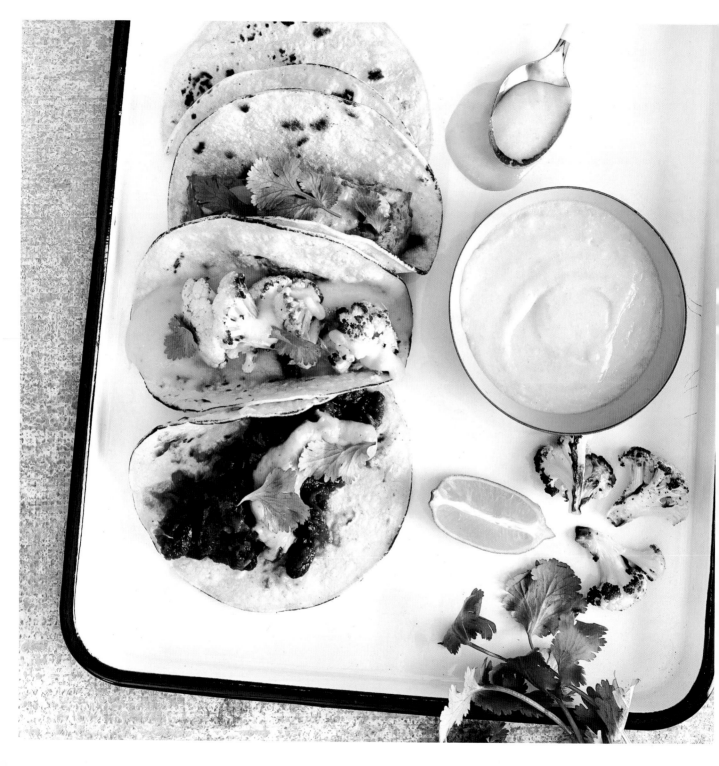

Pineapple-Habanero Bean Tacos

Makes 8 tacos

These tasty tacos have it all—some sweetness, some heat, and, yes, a heaping helping of plant-powered protein, thanks to the humble-but-mighty kidney bean.

1   tablespoon vegetable oil
1   medium-size red onion, finely chopped
1   teaspoon chopped garlic
1   (14-ounce) can tomato sauce
½   cup crushed pineapple in juice
1   habanero pepper, seeded and chopped
1   tablespoon soy sauce

1   tablespoon cider vinegar
1   teaspoon white miso paste
2   teaspoons freshly squeezed lemon juice
2   (15-ounce) cans kidney beans, drained and rinsed
8   corn tortillas, warmed

1 In a saucepan over medium heat, heat oil. Add red onion and sauté for 10 minutes, or until browned. Lower heat to low, add garlic, and sauté for 5 minutes, stirring occasionally. Add tomato sauce, pineapple with juice, habanero, soy sauce, and vinegar and simmer for 30 minutes. Turn off heat and add miso and lemon juice.

2 Using an immersion blender or standard blender, purée pineapple mixture. Return puréed pineapple mixture to saucepan and add beans. Simmer over low heat for 5 minutes. Serve warm with tortillas.

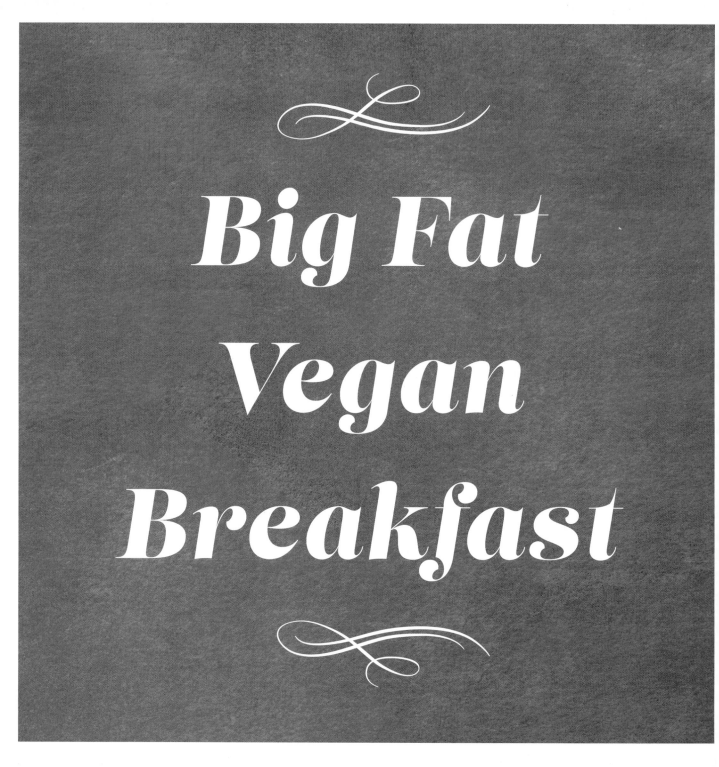

Day 4

If you want a real breakfast of champions, try one made without junky animal crap (and yes, there are vegan bagels and croissants and pancakes and scrambles and sausage).

Think back

to those days when you donned footed pajamas and rocked those crooked bangs, and your first thought when you woke up was, "Food!" For some of us, that was this morning. But assuming you were a kid, do you remember what your favorite breakfast was? An omelet and bacon? Froot Loops with milk and a cut-up banana? Pop-Tarts? Toaster Strudels? A pile of Bisquick pancakes? Soft-boiled eggs?

It's a funny thing—balancing the inherent nostalgia that we feel when we think of those early-morning meals we had growing up with the understanding we have now that the foods we were (and probably *are*) used to eating are laced with animal cruelty, and full of ingredients that our planet cannot sustain. Many people who first go vegan have the knee-jerk reaction of "Where does this leave me?" Add to that the blurry-eyed mayhem of the mornings, and veganism can feel hard to grasp for newbies—especially when you're trying to get out the door in a hurry. It doesn't have to be hard, though.

These days, in the rigmarole of our busy lives—whether we're balancing work or school or kids or dogs or just the hecticness of the modern-day morning—most of us have just a few go-to breakfasts on rotation. Oatmeal. Yogurt. A quick bagel. And since we are creatures of habit, the idea of changing up our morning routine to accommodate our plant-based diet can be perplexing at best, jarring at worst.

But the great news in all of that is that we are indeed creatures of habit, which means that with a few easy pivots—swap this for that, replace that with this—we can get into new habits more quickly than we can say "sunny-side up."

The other thing to keep in mind is that there is a vegan version of every single animal product out there. If you're taking notes, highlight that sentence, underline it, and put lots of stars and hearts next to it. It's worth repeating, and is the crux of what we're getting at here: there is a vegan version of literally *every* single animal product. That breakfast you're used to eating comes in a vegan version. The bacon and eggs, the yogurt, the French toast, the cereal, the milk, the omelet, the bagel and schmear, you name it: it comes vegan.

Sometimes when people go vegan, they bring a skepticism to the process that precedes all else, deciding ahead of time that the food is going to be gross, or it will be too hard to find vegan options on menus and in grocery stores. If you're a glass-is-half-empty (or half-full with cows' milk) kind of person, you're going to make it harder on yourself. So, let's make it easier.

First, remember that there is a vegan version of everything. Bear in mind that not every product is going to necessarily taste "exactly the same" as the animal-based foods you're used to. If you're inclined to think, "This is good, but it's *not the same*," remember that the point is not always to identically replicate (though oftentimes, the taste, texture, and flavor makeup is pretty spot-on); rather, it's to search for satisfaction and ring those same bells. And don't worry: you won't be skimping on taste. Never before has vegan food been so sophisticated, rich, complex, crave-worthy, and widely accessible as it is now. But as with anything else, you will need to try a few things to see what floats your fancy (did you really discover your favorite latte the first time you tried it?).

Keep in mind that just as with animal-based foods, there will be brands you like and brands you don't. No need to brush off veganism just because you don't like soy-based cheese; there's coconut-based or almond-based right around the corner.

It's also inspiring to remember how vastly different various cultures around the world look at breakfast. While in America, a typical breakfast might include eggs and bacon or pancakes and sausage, countries around the world have totally different takes on the morning meal. In China, that could mean vegetable soup, dumplings, fried sponge cake, or porridge. In India, a typical breakfast is *idli* and *sambar* (vegetable stew with steamed lentils and rice bread) or a dosa—a savory, crepelike dish made with fermented rice batter.

When you first try on vegan for size, think about what the vegan version of what you're currently eating could be. Focusing on that—and learning the plant-based equivalent of what you're used to—will be what 99 percent of those who are reading this should home in on. That means you replace your bacon with coconut bacon (try Googling a recipe, check out VegNews.com, or order Phoney Baloney's Coconut Bacon online); your meat sausage with tempeh or vegan sausage (try Gardein, Amy's, or Tofurky); your eggs with tofu or vegan eggs (try JUST Egg, Follow Your Heart VeganEgg, or Scramblit); and your cows' milk with any of the dozen plant-based milks out there (hemp, oat, peanut, almond, coconut, rice, banana, flax, cashew, pea, walnut, and good, old-fashioned soy). Trade out your dairy yogurts for vegan ones (from soy to cashew to almond), your butter for vegan butter (try Miyoko's European Style Cultured Vegan Butter or Earth Balance), and your cream cheese for the vegan version (there are tons, but we love Kite Hill, Daiya, and Follow Your Heart).

There are seriously so many vegan breakfast options out there that it is difficult to know where to start, which is why starting with what you currently eat—and veganizing it from there—is the easiest way to wrap your head around a diet change. Just as with nonvegan breakfasts, you can opt to get frozen or prepared versions, or you could easily put something together quickly from just a few items. Some great prepared breakfast options include MUSH Overnight Oats, Amy's Breakfast Scramble and Breakfast Burrito, or a banana (it even comes in its own convenient and compostable package!) with a single-serve packet of Justin's brand nut butter. Heck, pour some almond milk on your Cap'n Crunch (vegan, BTW) and you're good to go.

Some common vegan breakfasts include tofu scramble with toast; a breakfast burrito with refried beans, lettuce, tomato, and vegan cheese; veggie sausage or bacon; blueberry, apple, or carrot muffins; muesli or another dry cereal with fresh bananas and your favorite plant-based milk; chocolate chip pancakes; French toast; bagels with a vegan schmear or some blackberry jam; a robust fruit smoothie (with or without added greens); chilled overnight oats or hot steel-cut oats; nondairy yogurt with fruit and nuts; leftovers from the night before (cold vegan pizza for the win!); tempeh and vegetables; biscuits and gravy; a turmeric latte with some fresh fruit on the side; hash browns or golden potatoes with a chickpea-flour omelet; rice pudding; apple fritters with an espresso; freshly squeezed juice with a side of toast; or homemade waffles. That list could literally go on and on, since—say it with us—*there is a vegan version of every single animal product out there.*

While there is conflicting information out there on how critical breakfast is, for new vegans, it's superimportant to get all the taste, calories, healthy fat, and satisfaction possible, or you (or someone else) might feel the need to blame your new vegan lifestyle for any lull you feel from lack of eating. Avoid that by spending a little extra time planning your breakfasts, doing the proper grocery shopping and keeping a stocked fridge and freezer, and ensuring that any communal areas of your office offer vegan-friendly options (if your workplace has bagels every Monday, bring some vegan cream cheese and add it to the mix—and don't be surprised if it gets eaten first).

If at first you don't succeed, try another vegan option. Many vegans would say that breakfast is actually the easiest meal of the day, and regardless of whether you fancy yourself a cook or you are more of an instant-meal person, there's a foolproof way for every one of us to thrive on a vegan diet, starting the moment we wake up.

Light & Sweet

Coffee brings up so many emotions for so many people—so the idea of switching up your morning routine might feel jarring, especially if you're a cream-in-your-coffee person. Thankfully, just like coffee drinkers, plant-based creamers come in all types. Rest assured: there is a perfect vegan creamer for you. Here are five tried-and-true options guaranteed to bring on your morning (or afternoon or evening) coffee bliss.

CALIFIA FARMS

Addicted to a morning latte? Then you'll love the vegan creamers from Califia Farms. From straight-up creamer to flavored coffee add-ins (think: hazelnut and vanilla, along with coconut milk blends), this cool company will have you thinking outside the box (and outside the dairy) in no time.

MILKADAMIA

If you're nuts for macadamias, you need to try Milkadamia's equally rich creamer. Flavors come in Vanilla, Unsweetened Vanilla, and the ultimate indulgence—Macadamia Fudge.

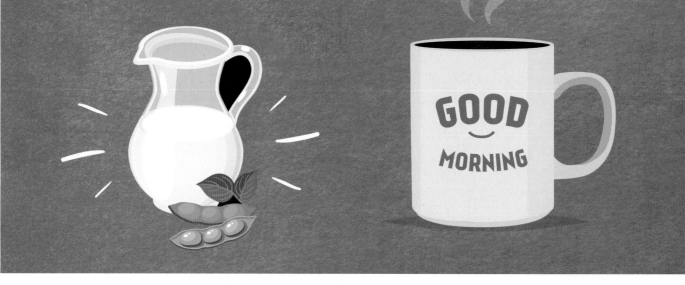

SILK

Before the almond, walnut, hemp, and coconut dairy-free options, there was Silk French Vanilla Soy Creamer, and it still reigns supreme. Watch it transform into the perfect creamer cloud as soon as it hits your coffee.

NUTPODS

Based in coconut, almond, and oats, Nutpods creamers are shelf-stable, sugar-free, supercreamy, and come in Hazelnut, French Vanilla, Caramel, and Original.

COFFEE-MATE

The most iconic coffee creamer company got with the program when it introduced its line of almond-based Natural Bliss creamers, available at many run-of-the-mill grocery stores. Get it in Vanilla, Hazelnut, or Caramel.

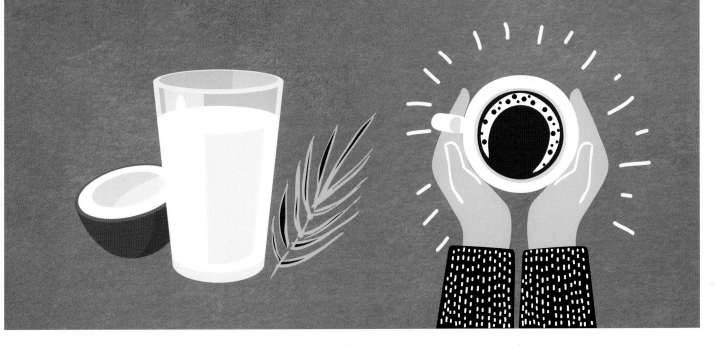

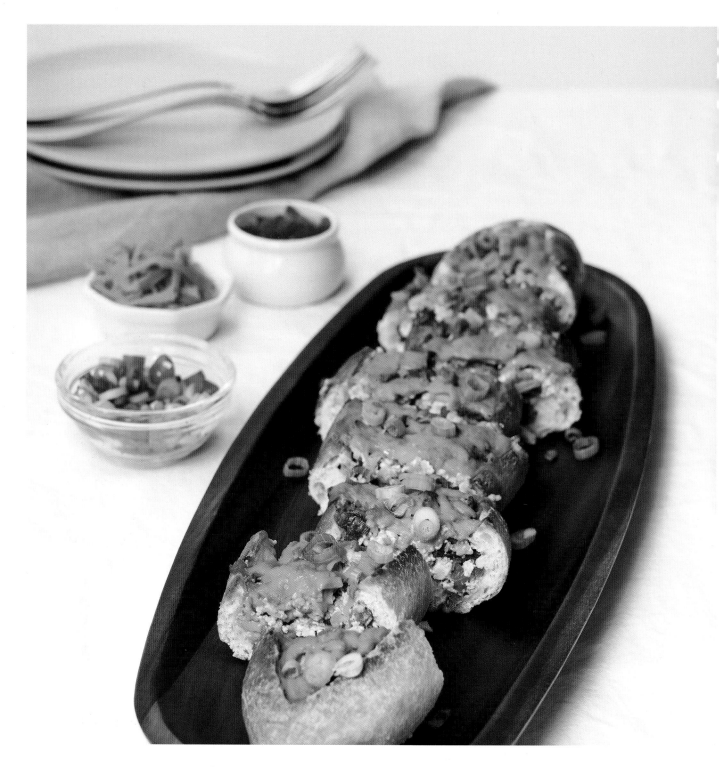

Bacon, Egg & Cheese Breakfast Boat

Serves 4

Filled with eggy scramble, bacon, sausage, and cheese, there's no doubt that this is the biggest, baddest, and best breakfast out there.

1   (26-inch) vegan baguette
¼   cup aquafaba (liquid from canned chickpeas)
½   (8-ounce) package extra-firm tofu, cubed
¼   cup seeded and diced red bell pepper
2   tablespoons plus 2 teaspoons sliced scallion
¼   cup chopped cooked vegan bacon
¼   cup chopped cooked vegan breakfast sausage

½   teaspoon salt
½   teaspoon granulated onion
½   teaspoon granulated garlic
½   teaspoon ground turmeric
½   cup plus 2 tablespoons shredded vegan Cheddar cheese
2   tablespoons vegan butter, at room temperature

❶ Preheat oven to 375°. Cut a rectangle along top of baguette without slicing to the bottom. Hollow out space for filling by removing interior bread.

❷ In a food processor, blend aquafaba for 20 to 30 seconds, or until white, frothy, and slightly thickened.

❸ Working in handfuls, squeeze tofu over sink to remove as much water as possible, and place in a large bowl. Crumble tofu to yield about 1 cup.

❹ To the tofu, add bell pepper, 2 tablespoons of scallion, bacon, sausage, salt, granulated onion, granulated garlic, turmeric, ½ cup of shredded Cheddar, and aquafaba. Mix to combine.

❺ Spread butter on inside of baguette and fill with tofu mixture. Place on a baking sheet and bake for 20 minutes. If baking sheet isn't long enough to hold baguette, place baguette directly on middle oven rack

❻ Remove from oven, and switch to HIGH broiler setting. Cut baguette into four equal pieces and top each with remaining 2 tablespoons of shredded Cheddar. Place on baking sheet and broil for 30 to 60 seconds, rotating occasionally, until cheese is melted. Slice into smaller pieces, garnish with remaining 2 teaspoons of scallion, and serve warm.

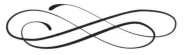

Finding Your Get-Up- and-Go

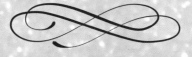

Day 5

*If you eat crap, you won't have enough energy, but if you eat a diet based on whole foods and healthy fats, **you'll be bouncing off the walls.***

Ever had a food

coma? You eat a giant piece of steak or other slab of meat and then suddenly you can't really move, and all you want to do is lie down. That makes sense, if you think about it. There's literally a dead piece of another living being now inside your body, and since food is fuel—and all of your energy is going into digesting that tough-to-break-down steak—you're going to feel depleted. Full stop. Animal-based foods will sit in your belly like a ton of bricks, take forever and a day to make it through you, and make it hell for you to poop (you know it's true).

Plant-based foods in their wholest forms, on the other hand—such as fresh vegetables, fruit, legumes, grains, nuts, and seeds—contain the necessary nutrients to help your body thrive, giving you the energy you need to be sustained throughout the day. They also contain fiber, which is key to a well-balanced diet—and helps you go to the bathroom, which

means you'll feel less lethargic and more energized. Whole plant foods also help to maintain steady glucose levels, so you won't crash as you would if you eat the aforementioned piece of dead animal.

This isn't rocket science. In fact, it's pretty simple. People who eat animal products don't automatically meet nutrient needs and can fall short on fiber as well as other compounds that many vegans consume on the daily. As for vegans, a well-planned diet can indeed meet all nutrient needs.

Food is our energy, and to thrive, we need a balanced and varied intake of hydration, carbs, proteins, good fats, vitamins, and minerals. Energy-wise, the most important thing to pay attention to is carbs. We literally run on carbohydrates (which is why overconsumption often results in fat storage).

Vegans who consume mostly whole foods not only eat large quantities of vegetables and fruit, but they also focus on good-for-you carbs, such as legumes and grains. Not only are these foods high in energy, but it's the slow-releasing type of energy. And though meat-eaters also eat these foods, we'd bet the farm that they most certainly don't eat as much as vegans.

When it comes to creating optimal energy, does milk really do a body good? Nope. Another energy-inhibitor is dairy, which can cause uncomfortable gastrointestinal (or digestive) issues, such as bloating, constipation, and gas, making you feel uncomfortable and sluggish. This is due to the fact that 65 percent of the global population is lactose-intolerant—meaning they do not have the lactase enzyme to break down the lactose sugars found in milk. Even those who are not intolerant may have a sensitivity to dairy, resulting in similar gastrointestinal discomfort and lethargy, which can take days to overcome.

So, where does all of this leave you? Plenty of vegan foods will help sustain you throughout the day and will give you a pick-me-up if you are starting to feel blah. Embrace a colorful diet, since a variety of vitamins, minerals, and nutrients are found through eating an array of fruit and vegetables. Start your day off with complex carbs, which are those found in whole grains, fruit, and vegetables.

And focus on fiber. Your digestion is slowed down by high-fiber foods, leveling off your blood sugar levels and keeping your energy level optimal. Greens, beans, whole grains, and nuts all provide a healthful dose of fiber.

Although there is definitely a place for mock meats and vegan versions of traditional, animal-based foods (the big silver lining here is that there is literally a vegan take on *every* animal product available), making the bulk of your diet focused on whole foods will help you thrive. If you're just starting your vegan journey, some power foods to focus on are lentils, almonds, quinoa, whole grains, and apples. These foods fill you up so that you won't be hungry throughout the day.

So, if you think you won't have any energy if you go vegan, think again. Those old myths that vegans only eat bean sprouts and slimy tofu, which precedes our patchouli ceremonies that we perform while wearing nonleather Birkenstocks and singing "Kumbaya" as a group before jumping on our bikes and heading to a nearby protest? They are just that—myths. There are a multiplicity of reasons to go vegan, but "I won't have enough energy" is not one of them. On the contrary: for those concerned about their energy levels, the very best thing to do is to ditch animal products for good.

10 Easy Ways to Boost Your Energy

Many new vegans naturally experience more energy once they give up animal products and embrace the power and nutritional properties of plant foods. Between that and getting enough z's, there are some easy pivots we can make to increase our energy levels and nip our fatigue in the bud.

1. **Drink enough water**—about a half-gallon each day.

2. **Steer clear of too many processed foods** and focus your diet on whole foods.

3. **Get out and move** every day, preferably in the sunshine.

4. Caffeine. It works. But **limit to one or two cups of coffee** or matcha lattes per day.

5. Make sure you're **taking your B$_{12}$**.

6. Have a **solid morning routine** that doesn't include staring at your phone or computer.

7. Have a **solid evening routine** where you can truly unwind (think: easy pajama-yoga with some chill background music).

8. **Step up your fruit and vegetable intake** by hiding them in unlikely foods, including smoothies, soups, and even brownies.

9. **Meditate** for at least a few minutes every day (download an app, such as Calm or Headspace, to help you out).

10. **Get up and stretch once an hour**, especially when you feel any kind of lull or need to change up the energy in the room.

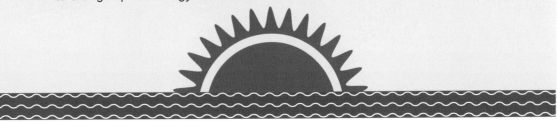

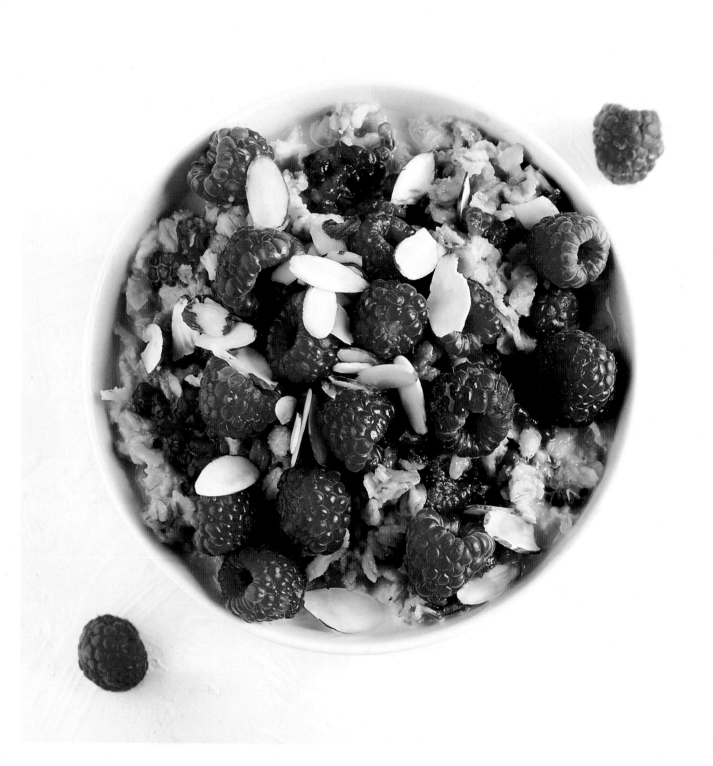

Raspberry Almond Butter Oatmeal Bowl

Serves 1

No more boring oatmeal here! This simple, filling bowl comes together in no time but provides a long-lasting boost of delicious energy.

1   cup water
⅛   teaspoon salt
¾   cup rolled oats
1   tablespoon coconut sugar
1   tablespoon almond butter

½   teaspoon pure vanilla extract
¾   cup raspberries
2   tablespoons unsweetened vanilla vegan milk
1   tablespoon slivered almonds

1 In a small saucepan over medium heat, combine water and salt, cover, and bring to a boil. Stir in oats, cover, and lower heat to medium-low. Cook, without stirring, for 5 minutes, or until oats are tender and excess water has evaporated.

2 Add coconut sugar, almond butter, and vanilla and stir. Transfer to a bowl, fold in raspberries, and top with milk and almonds.

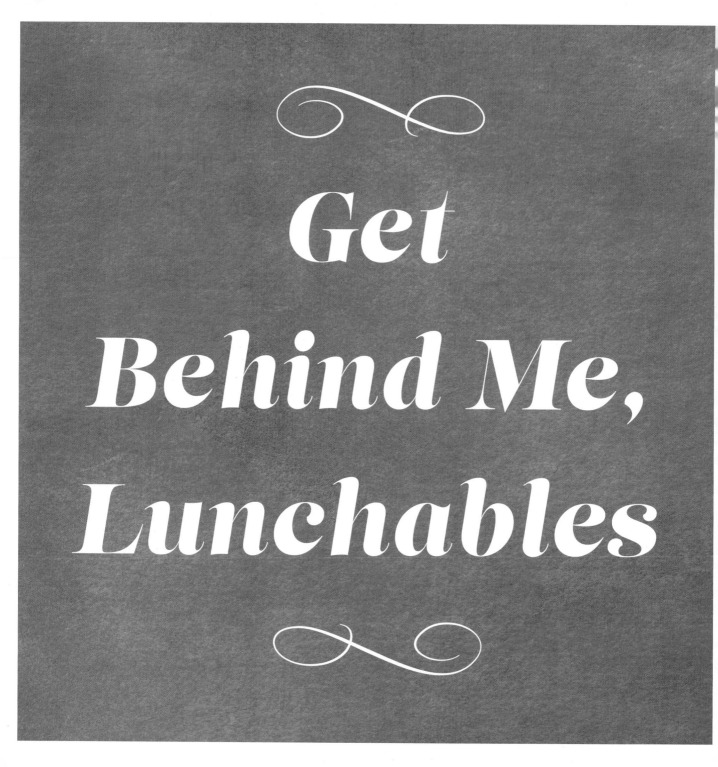

Get
Behind Me,
Lunchables

Day 6

We could fill this entire book with lunch options, and then create a multibook series. You will have more options than you know what to do with, but start here and we promise to keep it simple.

Seriously,

don't even think about touching our lunch. Whether you're an office worker and just looking for an excuse to escape from your sad cubicle, or a ten-year-old in math class staring down the clock as the minutes to freedom tick by, we all look forward to this midday meal break. As kids, the delightful sound of the recess bell meant time to catch up with friends, stick pencils in our nose, and fling little circles of ham from our Lunchables kits onto the ceiling of the cafeteria where they'd stay for the remainder of the school year. Or was that just us?

Fun fact: *lunch* is an abbreviation for the more formal northern English word *luncheon*, which was originally derived from the Anglo-Saxon word *nuncheon*—or *nunchin*—literally meaning "noon drink." And in medieval Germany, that referred to a midday snack of ale with bread, designed to break up the long, laborious days of harvesting and haying. It was the Middle Ages—long, long before the advent of Lunchables—that started to popularize lunch, thanks to pushing supper further back into the evenings, creating a gap in the middle of the day. And since toxic masculinity has roots that go *way* back, at that time, lunch was reserved for just the ladies (hence "the ladies who lunch"). In fact, the Prince of Wales once stopped in to join "the ladies" for lunch and was then endlessly taunted for being effeminate. This superweird gender role maladaption was thrown on its head in the nineteenth century when lunch became the norm, thanks to factory workers (men) who worked long hours, so factory-adjacent steakhouses started to provide mass-produced, meat-heavy meals.

These days, lunch can take many forms: from a festive holiday potluck to the stand-in-front-of-the-fridge-with-a-fork-eating-last-night's-leftovers lunch, which, admittedly, can be very satisfying. Although in many countries, lunch is the big meal of the day, for Americans, it's more often than not a quick thing to get people by between breakfast and dinner.

When you are new to veganism—especially if you live or work in places where the plant-based lifestyle is not yet the norm and there aren't too many veg-heads walking around—lunch can feel overwhelming. This might be a good moment to reiterate the fact that there's a vegan spin of every animal product out there, and with a few simple swaps, your go-to midday meals can very easily be pivoted to the plant-based equivalent.

To keep things doable, simply make a list of the lunches you usually eat, write out the specific ingredients that go into it, and then get yourself jazzed to find the vegan equivalent (it exists). A lot of this is going to be totally self-explanatory, and some of it will require a two-minute Google search. If you're used to eating ham and cheese, go for Tofurky Smoked Ham Style Deli Slices with Field Roast Chao Vegan Slices, with the usual schmear of mustard you like—and if you are a mayo person, opt for Vegenaise. There; you just re-created your sandwich. Now, add some easy veggie crudités, maybe a simple vegan ranch dip or nut butter to dip into, your favorite piece of fruit, and a dark chocolate square for dessert. If this is indeed your

jam, and a regular lunch choice for you, then make sure you prioritize getting these particular vegan essentials the next time you visit your grocery store. You don't need to spend hundreds of dollars and buy every vegan product ever made, to jump into veganism.

You'll also want to make sure to stock your fridge and cabinets with lunch-friendly vegan goods. This could include:

- ❑ a plethora of vegan condiments (many of the ones you already have—such as your basic ketchup and mustard—are already vegan, unless your mustard is honey Dijon)
- ❑ sauces (such as the supersimple marinara)
- ❑ dressings (go for Annie's Green Goddess dressing, or simple balsamic will also do)
- ❑ canned goods (don't forget the beans and chickpeas)
- ❑ vegetable stocks and bouillon cubes (though, in a pinch, you could always use water with spices added)
- ❑ pasta (you can go traditional whole wheat or opt for an odd but healthful bean pasta)
- ❑ whole grains
- ❑ nondairy staples such as sliced cheese, cream cheese, butter, milk, as well as vegan meats (trying every vegan meat will be your new favorite hobby)
- ❑ freezer essentials (get a few emergency frozen meals, such as burritos and pizza)

Keep it simple and remember that you really don't need to fill your kitchen with these staples all at once. It can indeed take a few trips to Trader Joe's to stock a kitchen this plentifully with vegan grub, and it's really not necessary to have absolutely everything from the get-go.

Even though most of us have just a few lunches that we eat on rotation—and it makes sense to start off your veganism by transitioning to the vegan equivalent of those foods instead of introducing completely foreign concepts—there are so many vegan lunch options that you could definitely eat a different lunch every day this year without repeating once. Some lunch ideas include vegan pesto pasta and broccoli (or pesto potatoes and broccoli); a rice, bean, and kale bowl with marinated tofu (if you have an air fryer, use it for making healthy tofu that has that "crispy fried" feeling without all the oil); avocado sushi; a smashed chickpea salad sandwich; a vegan bánh mì sub; Mexican quinoa; fried rice; and vegan Caesar salad with blackened tempeh.

That was really just an infinitesimal glimpse into what types of vegan lunches are possible. Just head to the aisle you would normally go to, and you'll usually find the vegan versions right alongside your former favorites. For example, nondairy yogurt is next to the dairy yogurts, frozen entrées are still in the freezer aisle, and you'll even find vegan burgers near the meat case. If you're still searching, the reliable refrigerated section with the good ol'
standby—tofu—will rarely let you down (though, on occasion, you will need to specifically seek out a "natural foods" aisle or fridge section).

And if you're still feeling nostalgic for those school days when you were busy blowing bubbles in chocolate milk and doing tradesies with your friends (your Fruit Roll-Up for my Reese's peanut butter cup!), then find hope in the fact that veganism is gaining momentum in schools. In New York City, all 1,700 public schools have adopted Meatless Mondays, with many schools offering vegan options. And in California, a bill was introduced into the legislature which, if passed, will provide funding to schools to increase the number of vegan options and plant-based milks on their menus. This kind of forward-thinking, vegan-friendly effort is becoming more and more commonplace.

When you think back to the roots of lunch—a meal of bread and ale that was created for "the ladies" to pass the time—it's pretty clear that things change and evolve for the better. Minds change, menus change, and meals change. If you need further evidence, look no further than Lunchables inventor Richard "Rody" Hawkins who, in 2018, raised $3 million to create the vegan meat company Improved Nature, featuring soy-based products such as Pork-Free Cutlets, Beef-Free Country-Fried Steak, and BBQ Boneless Chicken-Free Wings. These items, specifically created for food-service programs, are aiming to revolutionize, among other things, lunch. Or should we say, *nunch*.

Fast & Cheap, Like We Like It

No meatless restaurant just around the corner? No worries: Plant-based meals can be hacked from popular non-vegan restaurants with a little know-how. This list is constantly expanding, so keep an eye on VegNews.com for the latest.

AU BON PAIN

Many of the soups are vegan, including the Curried Rice and Lentil, Tuscan White Bean, French Moroccan Tomato Lentil, and Vegetarian Chili.

BURGER KING

Vegans can enjoy an Impossible Whopper (ask for it with no mayonnaise), a Garden Side Salad, fries, and hash browns. Hidden vegan treasures here are the French Toast Sticks and Dutch Apple Pie.

CHIPOTLE

The burritos, salads, and tacos can be made vegan by ordering with sofritas instead of meat; however, a sure bet is the Vegan Bowl made with sofritas, brown rice, black beans, romaine, tomato salsa, and corn salsa.

DEL TACO

Order the Avocado Beyond Tacos (vegan as is), the Beyond Tacos (ask for no cheese), or sub the meat in any item with Beyond Meat crumbles. Other options include the 8 Layer Veggie Burrito without cheese or sour cream; the ½ Lb. Bean & Cheese Burrito dairy-free; or the Signature Taco Salad sub Beyond crumbles, no cheese, and no sour cream. The crinkle-cut fries make the vegan cut, too.

DOMINO'S

Order the thin-crust pizza with no cheese and their original sauce; voilà, vegan.

EL POLLO LOCO

Get the BRC burrito sans cheese, with avocado or steamed broccoli as a side.

HARDEE'S/CARL'S JR.

No sacrifices here. Order the Beyond Famous Star burger without cheese or mayo. Round out the meal with the chain's vegan-friendly fries, hash rounds, or hash brown nuggets.

KFC

Colonel Sanders has partnered with Beyond Meat to veganize his "secret recipe." The Beyond Fried Chicken Nuggets with the Sweet N Tangy dipping sauce are vegan, and the Beyond Fried Chicken Boneless Wings can be veganized when ordered plain (the wing sauces contain honey). For sides, the corn on the cob, potato wedges, and salad are all vegan-approved.

SUBWAY

Enjoy a vegan version of a classic with the Beyond Meatball Marinara Sub. Ask for it on the Italian or 9-Grain bread and hold the cheese. For lighter options, try the Veggie Delite sandwich on Italian or sourdough bread or in a wrap. You can also create your own vegan-friendly footlong with the medley of fresh veggies and condiments on offer (hello, guac!).

TACO BELL

The chain recently launched a vegetarian menu, which includes such items as a 7-Layer Burrito, Black Beans and Rice, Spicy Tostada, and Power Menu Bowl, among others. Repeat after us: "Fresco Style," which is Taco Bell code for replacing the cheese, ranchero sauce, and sour cream with fresh pico de gallo. More Taco Bell Code: "Please replace the meat with beans." The chips, cinnamon twists, and Mexican rice are already vegan.

WHITE CASTLE

The oldest fast-food chain in the United States offers vegan hash browns, fries, and two plant-based burgers: a Veggie Slider and the Impossible Slider.

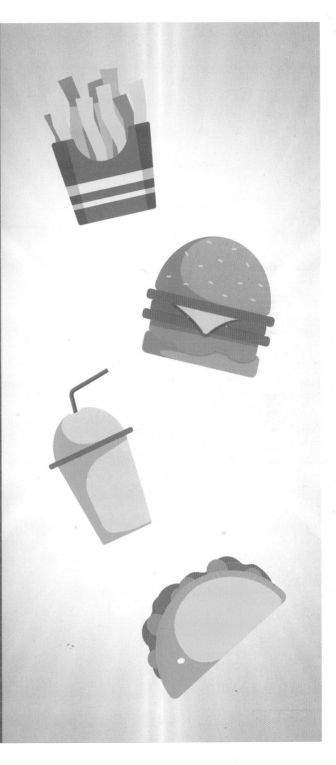

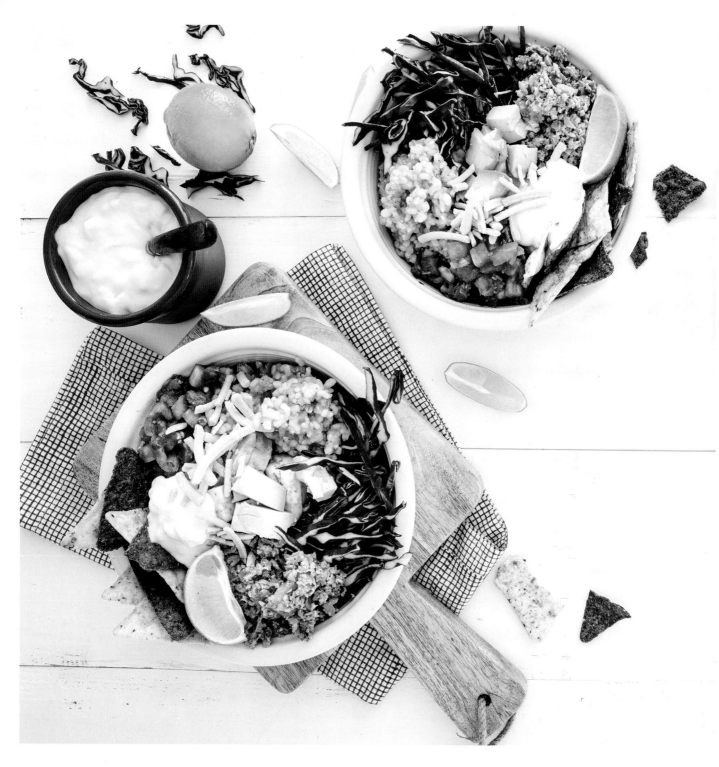

Spicy Vegan Chorizo Burrito Bowl

Serves 4

Chipotle's got nothing on you. This perfectly spiced, meaty homemade burrito bowl will be the envy of all your coworkers come lunch time. And best of all, there's no extra charge for guac.

Rice:
- 3 cups water
- 1½ cups short-grain brown rice
- ½ teaspoon garlic powder
- 1 teaspoon chili powder
- ¼ teaspoon cayenne pepper

Walnut-mushroom chorizo:
- 2 teaspoons safflower oil
- ½ medium-size yellow onion, finely chopped
- 2 garlic cloves, finely chopped
- 10 cremini mushrooms, finely chopped
- 1 cup toasted walnut pieces
- ¼ teaspoon cumin seeds
- ½ teaspoon salt
- ¼ teaspoon dried oregano
- ½ teaspoon ancho chile powder
- ½ teaspoon guajillo chile powder
- ½ teaspoon smoked paprika
- 3 tablespoons freshly squeezed lime juice
- 1 large tomato, deseeded and finely diced

Toppings:
- ½ cup pico de gallo or salsa
- ½ avocado, pitted, peeled, and diced
- ¼ cup pickled jalapeño slices
- 1 cup finely shredded purple cabbage
- 1 cup tortilla chips or strips
- ¼ cup vegan sour cream
- ¼ cup vegan cheese shreds

❶ **Prepare the rice:** In a large pot, bring the water to a boil. Add rice, garlic powder, chili powder, and cayenne. Cook, covered, for 30 to 35 minutes, or until tender.

❷ **Prepare the walnut-mushroom chorizo:** Heat a sauté pan over medium heat and heat oil. Add onion, garlic, mushrooms, walnuts, and cumin seeds and cook for 5 to 7 minutes, or until fragrant and golden.

❸ In a food processor or high-speed blender, combine cooked mushrooms, salt, oregano, ancho and guajillo chile powders, paprika, and lime juice and process until blended. Transfer mixture to a medium-size bowl, fold in tomato, and set aside.

❹ To serve, divide rice among four individual serving dishes. Top with walnut-mushroom chorizo, add your choice of toppings, and serve warm.

Vegan Food: It's Everywhere!

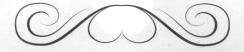

Day 7

*Trader Joe's, Walmart, Target, Safeway, Albertsons, Piggly Wiggly, you name it: **vegan foods are at literally every store.***

Repeat after

us: going vegan does not mean going broke. There is a huge misconception about this and it's just not true (it is also almost as eye roll–worthy as the protein question). Some of the healthiest, most mouthwatering foods just happen to also be the most budget-friendly.

Are you afraid that now is when we say "eat beans, and you'll single-handedly solve world hunger and create world peace" when you don't really want a bowl of beans for dinner—or ever, for that matter? The answer is a lot more nuanced than that. Although it's true that beans are healthful, cheap, eco-friendly, ethical, and can be prepared deliciously, when you're talking about being vegan on a budget, there's a lot more at play than beans.

Part of the reason why some people associate veganism with being expensive is because vegan specialty items—the processed, plant-based meats that are popping up more and more—often come with higher price tags than the cheap meat beside them on the shelves. These are premium products, and the hope is to get the price down as they scale up in quantity. It's that old supply-demand equation, which can be frustrating when you simply don't have the cash to buy the fancy thing, but many vegans opt for the fancy thing only on occasion (you can also make vegan meats at home, but that's next-level for some—try it in the *next* thirty days).

Keep in mind that the same could actually be said about meat, milk, and eggs. Animal products, too, come in so-called high-end, luxury items, which many people only get sometimes—the occasional "treat" to balance the more ordinary, day-to-day cabinet and fridge essentials. Yet luxury animal products don't often get a bad rap ("they're so expensive!"; "eating omni is way too pricey!") in the same way that the more luxurious vegan food options do. Your diet definitely doesn't need to revolve around imported vegan prosciutto, superfood powders, locally made cashew cheese spread, gourmet chocolate, and small-batch dips. You can be a well-fed vegan without even veering into those specialty items, if you so choose.

There's actually a cheap vegan section at every grocery store: it's called produce. Additionally, ethnic markets are inherently cheaper, and might also offer the cultural cues for communities of color who eat specific styles of food and want the vegan equivalent. Asian markets, for example, often offer big blocks of tofu—as well as miso, soy sauce, noodles, and rice—all at a fraction of the cost of what you'd likely find at Whole Foods. At Indian markets, you can often snag a great deal on chickpea flour, and at Latin markets, you'll want to stock up on tortillas.

A no-brainer for those on a budget is to also focus on the bulk bins. Not only can you buy exactly the amount you need of items such as pasta, flours, grains—and yes, beans—but you are saving money (not to mention the planet) by not paying for expensive and unnecessary packaging. If you have the time, making your own condiments, such as spice mixtures, salad dressings, mayonnaise, and even nut butters can save a lot of dough, too. So can comparison shopping to get the very best deals, taking

photos of items in your cabinets and fridge so that you don't waste money buying a second bottle of ketchup or a fifteenth container of baking powder, and Googling whether the store where you shop has any digital coupons you can quickly download.

But all of that takes time, and we don't always have the luxury of that. Worry not, because even if you are stretched thin for time (and change)—and if the nearest fancy-pants store is several towns away—you can still thrive as a vegan (without just eating bowl after bowl of rehydrated beans).

Staple foods you can pick up at most any grocery store include:

- ❑ fresh fruit and vegetables
- ❑ frozen fruit and vegetables for smoothies or stir-fries (don't knock frozen, as it carries nearly the same nutritional equivalent as fresh, and you can often find good sales)
- ❑ canned soups and sauces
- ❑ bread (many breads are vegan; just do a quick scan of the ingredients to make sure there's no random, unnecessary eggs, dairy, or honey lurking in there)
- ❑ nut butter
- ❑ oatmeal, brown rice, and pasta
- ❑ russet or sweet potatoes
- ❑ hummus
- ❑ nondairy milk (some stores offer great deals on house brand plant-based milks)
- ❑ olive oil
- ❑ mixed nuts

- ❑ salsa
- ❑ soy sauce (watch out for reduced-sodium soy sauce, which may contain lactic acid)
- ❑ condiments, such as mustard and ketchup
- ❑ baking supplies
- ❑ vegan snacks, including crackers and chips
- ❑ and yes, of course, beans (dried is cheapest, but canned is easiest and can also often be pretty inexpensive)

Then there's fast food. Although some readers have probably already scoffed, there are plenty of folks for whom fast food is the only option. If you're one of those people, it means you're superbusy—you work two jobs, or are a single parent, or student, or you simply live in an area where there are limited-to-no options when it comes to stores offering fresh produce and other healthful foods. These are known as food deserts, and they affect more than twenty-three million people in the United States. If you're one of them, then you know all too well that the struggle is real.

There are some serious issues at play here, and obviously there is no excuse for any individual to go without vegetables. But if you're reading this and you live in a food desert, or you're just too busy to cook right now, fast food might be your only option today. When it comes to going vegan, there's a silver lining here, since vegan options are becoming widely available at fast-food restaurants everywhere. In addition to the wide array of fast-food options at mainstream spots that we listed at the end of Chapter 6 (these include Burger King, Taco Bell, Carl's Jr., Del Taco, Chipotle, and many more), even the most unlikely culprits are starting to toy with the plant side. Sometimes, you just have to train yourself to look at menus differently to find the meat-free items.

Another reason that animal products are sometimes more available and less expensive than their plant-based counterparts is because of feed subsidies, which drastically reduce the price of meat. Basically, the vast majority of government-subsidized foods are meat and dairy, with fruit and vegetables receiving just a tiny portion of those subsidies. We'll get into this more in Chapter 22, but it's useful to keep in mind when rethinking your food choices as a whole.

For many, going vegan is easy-peasy, but it's important to remember that for some people—especially those in lower-income areas—there can be additional considerations that might make the logistics more time- or energy-consuming, initially.

For those whom this doesn't affect, it should not be used as an excuse—in fact, it's even more reason why we should go vegan, since at the heart of veganism is the spirit of using our privilege to stand for what is right for the environment, the animals, and ourselves. And for those of us who are in communities where the "rich-people stores" are only laughable and theoretical, veganism is still extremely doable—it just might require a bit more research into which stores and eateries near you carry what.

One last thing: you can eat beans if you want to.

Bargaining Power

Saving money isn't about sacrifice or sales; get all you need without forking over your paycheck with these simple hacks.

1. **Look high and low**—you'll find the best deals and more affordable brands on the top and bottom shelves.

2. Take advantage of **digital coupons**. Just download the store's app and scan in the savings.

3. Purchase your dry goods and nut butters from the **bulk bins**—less packaging means lower pricing.

4. Buy items with the **lowest unit price**, not retail price. You'll get more for what you pay.

5. Stay away from prepared produce and **chop your fruit and vegetables yourself**.

6 **Avoid the specialty products aisle** to steer clear of temptation and impulse buys. You don't need $20 worth of cacao nibs.

7 **Stock up in the frozen aisle.** Frozen produce is just as nutritious as fresh, and it's great to throw in a smoothie or stir-fry.

8 **Make a list of what you need** and stick to it.

9 Ask yourself, **"If it wasn't on sale, would I buy it?"** If the answer is no, leave it alone.

10 Give yourself a **maximum of 10 to 15 minutes** to make it to the cashier, so you only have time to grab the items you need.

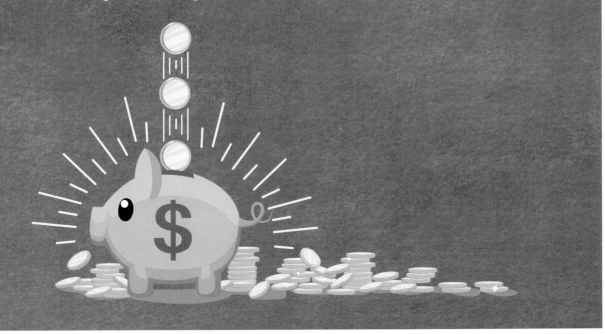

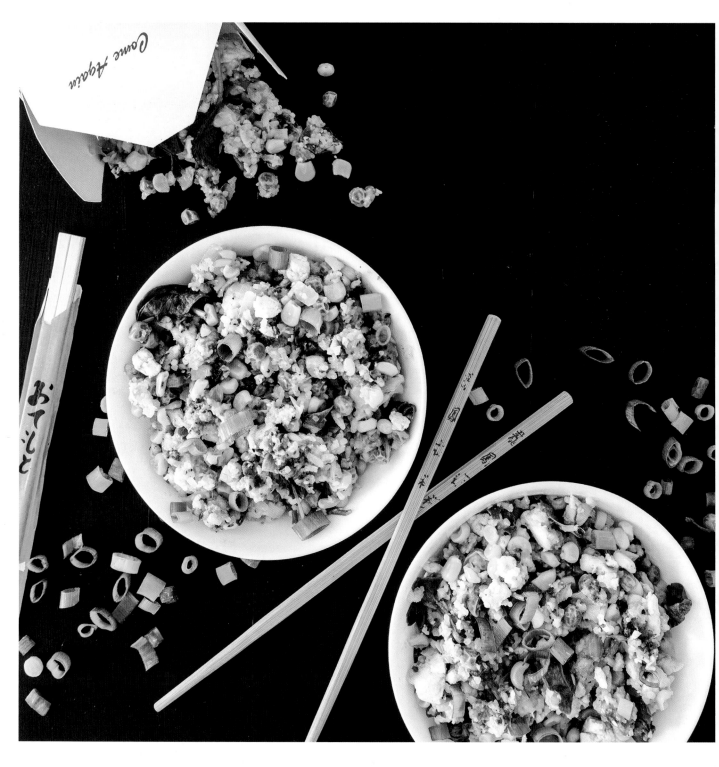

Chinese Vegetable Tofu Fried Rice

Serves 2

Who says a vegan meal needs to be expensive or hard to make? This takeout fakeout recipe requires just a few easy-to-access ingredients with a big-time yummy payoff.

1	tablespoon canola oil
1	(14-ounce) package extra-firm tofu, patted dry and crumbled
2	cups day-old cooked white rice
1	tablespoon toasted sesame oil
½	cup thinly sliced onion
½	cup thinly sliced scallions
4	garlic cloves, minced

2	teaspoons granulated garlic
2	teaspoons granulated onion
2	tablespoons soy sauce
¼	teaspoon freshly ground black pepper
1	cup frozen sweet corn
⅔	cup frozen petite peas
1	cup packed baby spinach, rinsed and drained

1 Over medium-high heat, heat canola oil in a large cast-iron skillet or wok. Add tofu and cook, stirring often, until golden brown, about 10 minutes. Microwave rice for 60 seconds on HIGH. Increase heat beneath skillet to high, add warmed rice, and cook, stirring and tossing, for 5 to 8 minutes, until rice is toasted and lightly golden.

2 Add sesame oil, onion, scallions, and minced garlic and cook, stirring gently, for 3 minutes, or until fragrant. Sprinkle granulated garlic and granulated onion over rice, tossing well. Add soy sauce, toss to coat, and sprinkle with pepper.

3 Add corn, peas, and spinach and stir until corn and peas are thawed and spinach is wilted, about 3 minutes. Remove from heat and serve immediately.

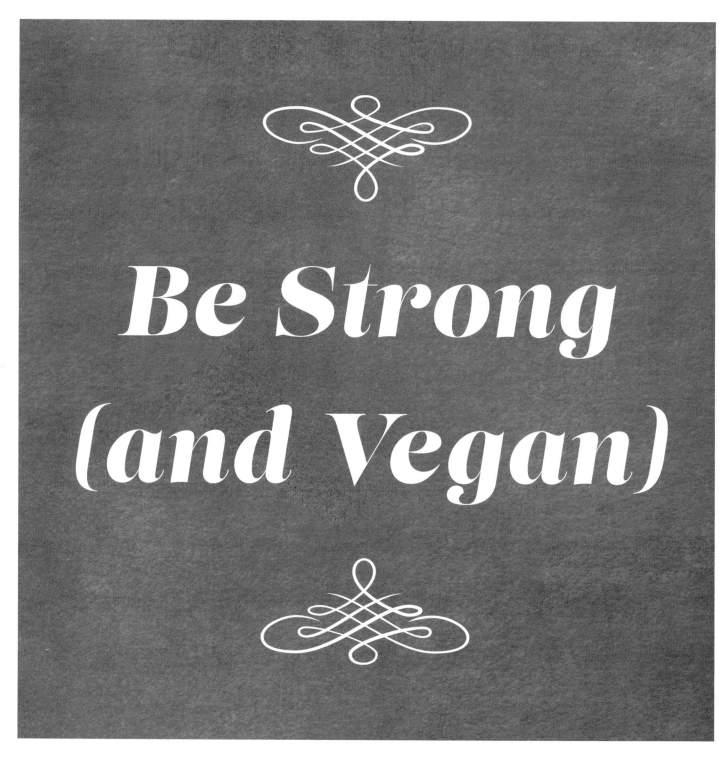

Be Strong (and Vegan)

Day 8

When you're talking about stepping up your fitness game, **the easiest and most effective way is to go vegan,** *whether you're into Krav Maga, SoulCycle, yoga, CrossFit, ballet, jujitsu, curb-hopping, or whatever.*

When you think

of fitness, what comes to mind? A ripped weight-lifter flaunting their perfectly chiseled eight-pack? A woman in a sleeveless tee shooting hoops at the park? A person in dolphin shorts rollerblading on the boardwalk of their mind? Whatever your brand of fitness—from yoga to AcroYoga to aerial yoga to hot yoga (so many yogas!), to CrossFit, Soul-Cycle, parkour, swimming, figure skating, Jazzercise, pole-vaulting, or pole dancing—you can do all of it and then some while being completely fit and entirely vegan. Yes, indeed—in case you haven't been paying attention thus far—you can be fit and healthy while eating nothing but plants.

Three Little Words

Whether your athleticism is old hat and you have the medals to prove it, or you've just loaded up the "Couch to 5K" app on your phone and you're ready to give it a go—there are three very important words you'll want to familiarize yourself with: carbs, fats, and protein (just bear with us here). Yes, we need these macronutrients—as does every other human being—but when you're pushing your body to do more than just sit there, it needs a bit more of these things.

Carbs give you energy during your workout—that goes for everything from basketball to ultrarunning. In fact, carbohydrates break down into glucose, which is the most efficient form of energy during exercise—and athletic performance is all about efficiency. If you're working out for more than an hour, consuming carbs during your workout can help fight off fatigue (we're not saying you should eat a bagel midrun, but popping a delicious date or two can definitely give you a second wind—get that bagel and vegan schmear later). You don't have to eat before a workout, but some swear that a banana or piece of toast with peanut butter succeeds in giving them that boost they need (and preworkout fuel is really up to personal preference). Consuming carbs with a bit of protein has been shown to deliver a steadier stream of glucose to the muscles, as opposed to consuming carb-rich foods without much protein (such as eating a banana with peanut butter versus shooting an energy gel—the first will give you sustained energy, whereas the gel will just give you a quick and immediate burst).

Fats. Like carbs, fats are a form of energy. Think of fats as your backup reserve. During low- to moderate-intensity workouts, our body can transition to burning fat as its fuel source, since we don't need the energy as immediately (that's because it takes longer to convert fat to fuel, in comparison to carbs). Just don't rely on an avocado to push you during that one-rep bench press or 60-second CrossFit burpee challenge; carbs are the go-to for high-intensity efforts. Also, when your glycogen stores run out, your body turns to fat to burn, as it's easier to convert to energy than protein. If you run out of carbs and fat, your body starts to go for the protein in the muscles, which means it's eating itself. Don't do that.

Protein. It's true that protein helps build muscle, but it doesn't have to come from an animal to give you power. While the daily recommended amount is 0.36 grams of protein per pound of body weight, it is recommended that athletes take in a bit more. Generally, 0.54 grams per pound of body weight for endurance athletes and 0.73 grams per pound of body weight for strength athletes is the golden rule. And (this is important) more protein does not mean more muscle; your body can only absorb so much. It's important to eat a snack or balanced meal postworkout that contains protein to stimulate efficient muscle synthesis. You've just broken down muscle fibers, and you need the amino acids in protein to help repair those fibers (and in doing so, you build muscle). Enjoy a postworkout smoothie with leafy greens, a bit of fruit for a carbohydrate kick, or a tablespoon or two of nut butter or hemp seeds for a protein punch. Even something as simple as a glass of soy milk will do the trick. Oatmeal, hummus and carrot sticks, tofu scramble . . . you will not run out of options.

Micronutrients & Antioxidants. For extra credit (You: "Wait, this is a quiz?!"), let's talk micronutrients and antioxidants. You don't get many of these beneficial compounds with a chicken's breast or a whey protein shake (*no whey!* . . . sorry). However, plant foods are full of these "secret weapon" nutrients that help your body perform at its optimum best. Take berries, for example. They're full of antioxidants that help fight inflammation and speed recovery. Whether you're a barre enthusiast, obstacle course racer, or die-hard weekend warrior cyclist, the goal is to reduce your body's inflammation so you can recover and get back at it the next day so that you can do more pliés, scale more muddy walls, or cycle up that mountain faster. Another example is potassium. This nutrient doubles as an electrolyte and helps prevent muscle cramping. Athletes don't need to rely on sports drinks or gels to replenish their electrolyte storage—such foods as potatoes and white beans are terrific sources of potassium. Essentially, plants help speed recovery by fighting inflammation, and every single athlete can benefit from this (but you already knew that—so, congratulations: you aced the quiz you didn't know you were taking!).

A Word (or 250) on Strength Training

Right next to myths about protein and gluten (see page 99), there's this idea that vegan = weak. But just Google "vegan bodybuilders" and then tell us whether the musclemen and women in the images look weak to you (or just skip Googling it entirely and trust us that you would not want to get on their bad side anytime soon). Strength training comprises many things: you've got weightlifting and powerlifting (different techniques to lift a helluva lot of weight) as well as sculpting, maintenance, and moderate exercise to gain lean muscle mass (think of that woman shooting hoops whose arms made you dribble your oat milk latte). If you're not gaining that muscle mass and you want to, up your daily caloric intake by 500 to 1,000 of delicious and wholesome vegan calories.

Beyond calories, vegan strength trainers probably get The Protein Question more than anyone else. While the Institute of Medicine (which sets the Recommended Dietary Allowance, or RDA) actually has no statement recommending athletes take in more protein, the Academy of Nutrition and Dietetics, the American College of Sports Medicine, and Dietitians of Canada published a joint position paper underlining the value of increasing protein intake if you're an athlete, as well as paying attention to the timing of the protein intake.

Although protein is available in most food, some particularly high vegan sources that many ripped athletes incorporate into their days include legumes (lentils, chickpeas, and yes, peanuts), seitan, tofu, quinoa, and sometimes supplements such as protein powders. (If bodybuilding is your thing, you should also be sure to have enough high-quality fat, and omega-3 and omega-6 fatty acids.)

Resistance exercise also requires carbohydrate intake (this will happen naturally as long as you're getting your daily dose of protein and fat intake from whole food sources) as well as vitamins and minerals (especially B_{12}, calcium, iodine, and vitamin D).

Food, Glorious Food

You don't have to be an award-winning cook to make athlete-friendly recipes. Such websites as VegNews.com (yeah, baby!) and NoMeatAthlete .com are loaded with nutrient-dense, performance-optimizing recipes that even someone with only a pan, a spatula, and maybe a blender (even if it was your mom's in the '80s and is still somehow kicking) can master. From a plethora of simple smoothies (with or without added protein powder), homemade granola bars (they are way easier, yummier, and less hippie-dippy than you think), to carb-heavy loaded sweet potatoes, there are endless ways of bettering your fitness, starting with your grub. Healthy fats (such as avocado, nuts, and seeds), wholesome grains (such as quinoa, brown rice, and millet), and plenty of vegetables mean that you will stay fuller

The Next Generation of Athletes

Vegan athletes of all stripes are illustrating that the easiest way to step up their game is by eating plants. These vegan powerhouses are sweeping the competition and shattering the protein myth, proving that you can get ripped and chiseled—and go fast and long—without eating any animal products.

ALEX MORGAN

Sport: Soccer

Reason for going vegan: A dog-lover for life, Morgan looked down at her pooch and made the connection, realizing that there is no difference from the animals we love and the animals we eat.

Go-to power-packed meal: Mexican-inspired, plant-based bowl

Athletic accolades: 2012 Olympic gold medalist; 2015 FIFA Women's World Cup Champion; 2019 FIFA Women's World Cup Champion

Wise words: "I am passionate about giving animals a voice. I even adopted a vegan diet, because it didn't feel fair to have a dog I adore, and yet eat meat all the time."

NIMAI DELGADO

Sport: Natural bodybuilding

Reason for going vegan: Raised vegetarian, Delgado ditched all animal products after doing his research and realizing that animals in the dairy and egg industries are treated just

and more energized for longer periods of time. It also means you'll be less grumpy, and there's pretty much nothing worse than a grumpy athlete.

As you're improving your performance and experimenting with veganism, you might want to start to track your journey, your body, and your results; it's the easiest and often most useful type of self-accountability. No need to invest in a fancy workout journal; a regular cheap notebook from the dollar store will do just fine (we like the ones with unicorns on the cover, but *you do you*). Map out how many days a week you are planning to exercise, what you eat before and after you do, and how your energy shifts. If you're feeling low on energy, check in with yourself to make sure you're eating enough calories. Whole, plant-based foods tend to be lower in calories than animal-based foods, so you might be eating less without realizing it. If that's the case, as poorly as those raised for meat. Once he saw an improvement in his athletic recovery and decrease in inflammation, he knew he was never going back.

Go-to power-packed meal: Buddha bowl with tofu, mixed greens, chickpeas, avocado, and sweet potato

Athletic accolades: Won his first bodybuilding competition as a vegan in 2016; International Federation of Bodybuilding and Fitness (IFBB) Pro; graced the cover of *Muscle & Fitness Magazine*, April 2018

Wise words: "Ditching dairy allowed me to recover quicker which allowed me to get into the gym more frequently which allowed me to make bigger gains, faster, overnight almost."

HOLLY MATTA

Sport: CrossFit

Reason for going vegan: A self-proclaimed "carnivore-turned-herbivore," Matta went vegan to reach her health and fitness goals.

Go-to power-packed meal: Baked apple pie chia pudding

Athletic accolades: 6x competitor in the CrossFit Open; 7x Regional competitor in the CrossFit Games; Ranked #37 in the world for Individual Women at the 2013 CrossFit Games

Wise words: "I want to be as healthy as I can and live as long as I can for my family. I want to inspire others to ditch dairy and meat to feel their very best and to debunk all the things out there saying you need dairy and meat to get your protein."

comfort foods, such as seitan, tempeh, nut butter smoothies, and pasta dishes can help make up the difference. If you're really into numbers, you can track your sleep, too (Fitbit is great for this, and a lot cheaper than some other smart watches); make sure you're getting at least seven hours a night, no matter what (that means you have to turn off *Real Housewives* at a reasonable hour, friend).

Truly, absolutely, and without question, vegans are strong in every way—and athletes have definitely gotten that memo, because more and more movers and shakers are realizing that when it comes to optimal athletic performance, animal products only hold you back. Are you picking up what we're putting down yet? These professionals are all the proof you need that plants contain the most powerful fuel there is.

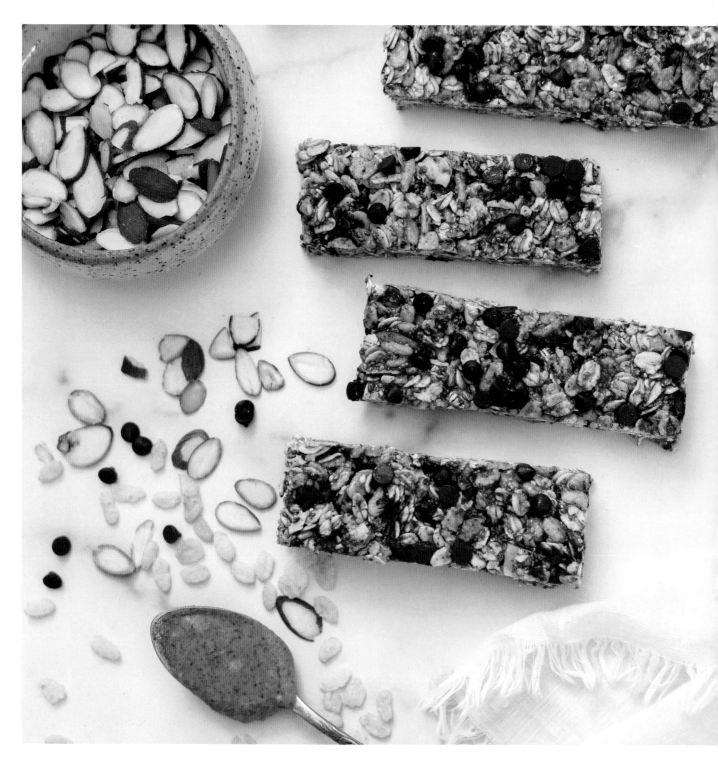

Chocolate Almond Oat Power Bars

Makes 12 bars

These wholesome bars are packed with almond butter, chia seeds, and hemp seeds and given a sweet finish with chocolate chips and a kiss of maple syrup. Bonus: there are 4.3 grams of protein per bar!

½   cup sliced almonds or finely chopped whole almonds
1½   cups rolled oats
1   cup puffed rice cereal
3   tablespoons chia seeds
2   tablespoons hulled hemp seeds
½   teaspoon ground cinnamon

¼   teaspoon salt
½   cup brown rice syrup
¼   cup smooth almond butter
1   tablespoon pure maple syrup
1   teaspoon pure vanilla extract
1   vanilla bean pod, seeds scraped and reserved
¼   cup mini vegan chocolate chips

❶ Preheat oven to 325°F. On a baking sheet, spread out almonds and toast for 10 to 12 minutes, or until lightly golden. In a large bowl, stir together toasted almonds, oats, cereal, chia seeds, hemp seeds, cinnamon, and salt.

❷ In a medium-size saucepan over low heat, whisk together brown rice syrup, almond butter, and maple syrup until smooth. Increase heat to medium and bring to a low simmer while stirring. Remove pot from heat after 1 to 2 minutes.

❸ Into brown rice syrup mixture, whisk vanilla extract and vanilla bean seeds. Let sit for 1 minute to cool. Pour syrup mixture over dry ingredients, stirring with a metal spoon until well combined. Let sit for 1 minute to cool, then stir in 3 tablespoons of chocolate chips.

❹ Line a 9-inch square pan with parchment paper. Spoon mixture into prepared pan and gently spread with damp hands until it fills pan. Sprinkle with remaining tablespoon of chocolate chips and lightly press down on mixture until even.

❺ Place pan, uncovered, in freezer to chill for 10 to 15 minutes, or until firm. Cut into bars, using a pizza slicer or serrated knife. The bars can be wrapped in plastic wrap, then placed in a zip-top bag and stored in a sealed container in the refrigerator for up to 1 week or in the freezer for up to 1 month.

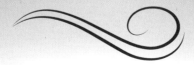

For All the Salad-Haters

Day 9

You can be vegan and never eat a salad again. You can actually be vegan and never eat vegetables (but we don't recommend it).

Many people

equate a salad with rabbit food, and sometimes for good reason. Bunnies also love to eat basil, bok choy, carrot tops, collard greens, lettuce, watercress, and other fresh fruit and vegetables that some vegans consider central to their diet. Looks like Bugs was definitely onto something.

On the other hand, many people's initial response when you ask them what a salad is usually falls somewhere between cold iceberg lettuce with mealy tomatoes and maybe some bitter vinegar or gloppy dressing (and sad, stale croutons). Yet salads can more closely resemble robust bowls. Imagine an array of cooked greens; crispy protein, such as baked tofu or tempeh; a rich tahini sauce dressing; and even the sweet finish of crispy, succulent apple slices with a sprinkling of crunchy, toasted walnut crumbles.

And if that's still too salady for you, you can definitely leave the lettuce for the rabbits. There are still endless ways to consume a fresh, healthy vegan diet that's good for you, the planet, and the animals who are no longer part of your meal. Dinner as a vegan can be full of rich, varied, abundant, healthful, filling food—no cold lettuce required.

By now, your fridge and pantry are probably pretty well stocked. So, next, if you have the means, you might want to consider investing in one or a few kitchen appliances. We'll lay out some possibilities for you here, but don't think that you absolutely have to have these to thrive as a vegan; you don't. Literally, all you really need is a pot and maybe a pan. The rest is (mushroom) gravy—you can either get it or not get it, add it to your birthday list or wedding registry or make a passive-aggressive hint to your parent or spouse about how much you want it, or simply throw it into your Amazon shopping cart and then stare at it while sipping cheap wine and crying real tears.

That said, lots of vegans swear by a high-powered blender, such as a Vitamix (no, not every blender is created equally, and Vitamix is among the best out there); a simple steamer (consider a bamboo steamer basket, which allows you to steam in multiple layers); an air-fryer (not to be dramatic but this will basically permanently transform your life for the better); a food processor (it's a good old standby for a reason); a pressure cooker (prioritize this if you are impatient and like immediate gratification); a slow cooker (consider this your at-home cook, since all you have to do is throw a few ingredients in it in the morning, and when you get home from school or work, your dinner will be ready for you—*voilà!*); a spiralizer (did you know that you can magically turn squash or zucchini into pasta?); and a cast-iron skillet (it doubles as a free weight). Any of these will help you feel empowered to really conquer dinner (or any meal, really), but again, you don't absolutely need them any more than you need to eat rabbit food for din-din.

Because so many of us wince at the idea of change, a lot of people's first reactions when they go vegan is, "What will I eat for dinner?" You already know by now that the answer is to simply have the vegan version of what you already like.

The billions and billions of online resources that have been created since the internet's existence will come in handy right now, as you start to tackle this fun puzzle of finding the plant-based version of whatever your favorite suppertime meal is—such as quiche (tofu—instead of eggs—can make a mean one, as can an egg replacer product, such as VeganEgg or Scramblit), chicken piccata (try seitan piccata instead and thank us later), or pasta (this is perfect for lazy or busy people, as a huge amount of canned or shelf-stable pasta sauces—beginning but certainly not ending with marinara—are inherently vegan). And, of course (cue the shameless plug), a subscription to VegNews magazine—plus regularly visiting VegNews.com—will help you immensely on your way, as we publish the best recipes, the best insights, the best news, and the best of everything vegan. Say it with us now: there is a vegan version of every single animal product out there. Say it again. Say it one more time.

Transition foods—vegan meats and cheeses—will be your BFF as you start and stay on your vegan journey. Beyond veganizing the foods you're used to eating, you might consider any of the following of these for dinner:

❏ macaroni and cheese (you can, in fact, get the boxed stuff if you want, but you might want to experiment with making a creamy cheese sauce in the blender, or see page 63 for our recipe)

❏ vegetable stir-fry over soba or udon noodles (watch out for instant cup–style noodles that may contain lactic acid)

❏ a hearty greens, beans, and grains bowl made with—you guessed it—your favorite kind of greens, beans, and grains accompanied by chopped sweet potato and drizzled with tahini with a generous dash of vegan Parm to finish

- [ ] any kind of pasta, such as butternut squash linguine or gnocchi with vegan pesto pasta (Trader Joe's has a ready-made vegan kale pesto that might quickly become your favorite staple)
- [ ] vegetable paella
- [ ] a veggie burger with a side of fries and a vegan coleslaw (play with all the different brands of burger patties—and remember that you could go traditional "beefy" or old-school black bean patty)
- [ ] West African peanut soup (surprisingly simple to make)
- [ ] tacos (honestly, the sky's the limit here—from grilled asparagus and shiitake to crumbled vegan beef with charred greens)
- [ ] squash-lentil stew (if you make it in a slow cooker, it'll be ready when you get home)
- [ ] rainbow veggie-kebabs with tofu or faux sausage
- [ ] peanut, edamame, and noodle salad (sorry to use the s-word, but c'mon!)
- [ ] a vegan meatball and cheese sub (to remember your real or imagined Italian roots)
- [ ] melty vegan grilled cheese with tomato soup (we all could use a fifth grader–approved dinner from time to time)

The list goes on and on (and on and on and on). We could literally fill up this entire book with just one giant paragraph pointing out dinner possibilities. Are you hungry yet?

Veganism is a lot of things, but "difficult" doesn't have to be one of them. A lot of the fear that people bring to the table has to do more with the discomfort that comes with changing any habit, and with worrying whether those around you will be judgmental or put off. One of the best ways to advocate for veganism is through sharing delicious food, so even if your social circles don't want to make the full commitment to going vegan, they'd likely be happy to help share a meal with you. Once you bite the bullet—and the veggie burger—you'll find that it's a lot easier than you thought. Bring a vegan cheese plate to a party, and we're telling you, that shit will disappear.

The word *vegan* has become full of so much hype, and that can feel intimidating—especially if you don't have a vegan or vegan-friendly support system intact. The only way over that hump is over that hump, and the fact that vegan food is more delicious and accessible than ever before will make this a really easy transition for you. You'll have a few hiccups along the way for sure, where you accidentally get silken tofu (great for puddings, not so much for anything else) instead of extra-firm, but you'll get through it. Let the unique blend of the mystery and familiarity of vegan food guide you here, and you'll quickly be old hat. Once you rethink your food choices and lean into your veganism, who knows? Maybe next you'll start to rethink your opinion on salads.

8 Salads You Didn't Realize Were Salads

Don't worry; there's not a single leaf of lettuce in these hearty meals!

1 SOBA NOODLE SALAD

Simply cook vegan soba noodles according to package instructions, drain, and chill while you dice up some veggies and thaw some frozen edamame. Toss the veggies, edamame, and noodles together with a store-bought peanut sauce and dig in with those chopsticks. Extra hungry? Chop up a square of baked tofu (try Wildwood or Nasoya brands) and throw these flavorful protein-packed cubes into the mix.

2 CHICKPEA TUNA SALAD

Sub fork-mashed chickpeas for the tuna, then add the ingredients you typically use (just swap out the mayo for vegan mayo, such as Vegenaise). Our favorite combo includes mashed chickpeas, a squeeze of vegan mayo, a squirt of mustard, finely chopped red onion, a few heaping spoonfuls of relish, and a sprinkle of nori or dulse flakes for fanciness and a fish-free fishy taste.

3 TOFU EGG SALAD

Similar to chickpea salad, you really only need to sub out one ingredient—the egg—and use vegan mayo instead of traditional. Try crumbling firm tofu and mixing it with mayo, a bit of mustard, chopped celery, and a pinch each of salt, pepper, garlic powder, turmeric, and nutritional yeast. Slather between two slices of bread, and you just turned your salad into a sandwich.

4 WATERMELON SALAD

Cube some watermelon, toss with vegan feta (make your own from tofu if you're feeling like a

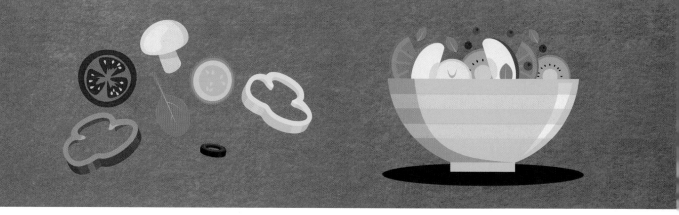

vegan Julia Child, or order some Urban Cheese-craft Dairy-Free Feta Mix if you're feeling lazy), add a flourish of chopped fresh mint or basil, and finish with a drizzle of balsamic vinegar.

5 PASTA SALAD

To veganize your favorite recipe, just omit the cheese or sub in a vegan cheese alternative, such as Violife. This is a great clean-out-the-fridge salad, and it keeps for a few days.

6 POTATO SALAD

Just trade the mayo in your favorite potato salad for a vegan one, and you're golden. If your family's potato salad includes bacon, throw in some store-bought vegan bacon (such as the Herbivorous Butcher Maple Glazed Bacon or Lightlife Smart Bacon).

7 CAPRESE SALAD

Slice up some tomatoes (heirloom will offer the most flavor, but it's fine if you're using good old-fashioned Roma or beefsteak tomatoes), layer with store-bought vegan mozzarella (trust in Miyoko's brand), scatter a few basil leaves on top, add a pinch of salt, and drizzle with balsamic.

8 CRUCIFEROUS SALAD

Simply use a food processor or hand grater to chop up equal parts broccoli and cauliflower florets into tiny quinoa-size pieces. Then, shred in about half that amount of grated carrot. Add a handful of raisins and a few chopped walnuts if you're a crunch fanatic. Toss it all in a big bowl with a drizzle of maple syrup, a squeeze of lemon juice, and salt, pepper, and cayenne to taste.

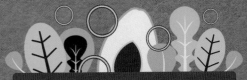

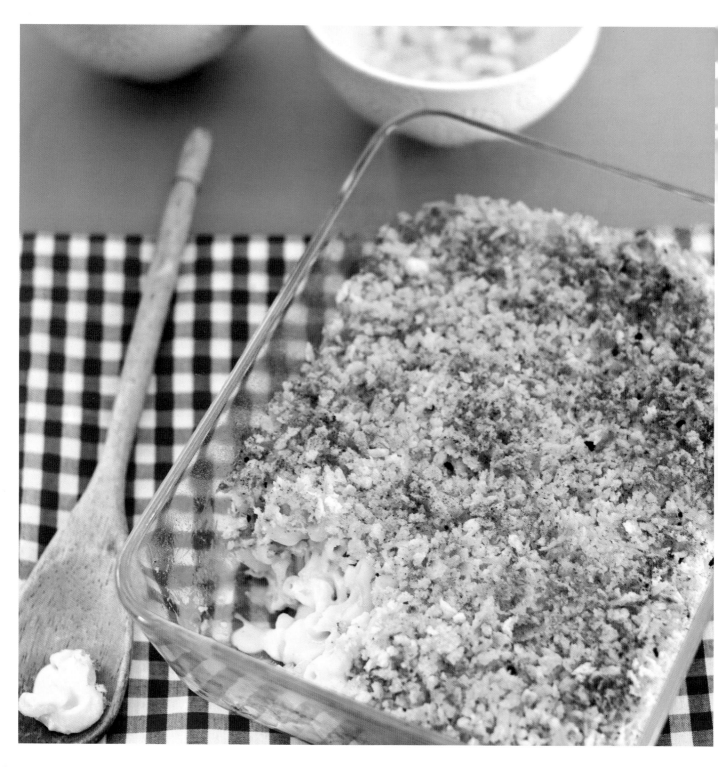

Best Ever Mac & Cheese

This vegan mac & cheese created by Allison Rivers Samson is the absolute best on the planet. Our tip? Double the sauce and use rigatoni or cavatappi pasta to get even more cheese per forkful.

4 quarts plus 1 cup water	⅓ cup chopped onion
1 tablespoon plus 2 teaspoons salt	¼ cup raw cashews
8 ounces macaroni pasta	¼ teaspoon minced garlic
4 slices vegan bread, torn into large pieces	¼ teaspoon Dijon mustard
⅓ cup plus 2 tablespoons vegan butter	1 tablespoon freshly squeezed lemon juice
2 tablespoons chopped shallot	¼ teaspoon freshly ground black pepper
1 cup peeled and chopped red or yellow potatoes	⅛ teaspoon cayenne pepper
¼ cup peeled and chopped carrot	¼ teaspoon paprika

1 In a large pot, combine 4 quarts of water and 1 tablespoon of salt and bring to a boil. Add macaroni and cook until al dente. In a colander, drain pasta and rinse with cold water. Set aside.

2 In a food processor, make bread crumbs by pulverizing bread and 2 tablespoons of vegan butter to a medium-fine texture. Set aside.

3 Preheat oven to 350°F. In a saucepan, combine shallot, potato, carrot, onion, and remaining cup of water and bring to a boil. Cover pan and simmer for 15 minutes, or until vegetables are very soft.

4 In a blender, combine cashews, remaining 2 teaspoons of salt, remaining ⅓ cup of vegan butter, garlic, mustard, lemon juice, black pepper, and cayenne and blend. Add softened vegetables and cooking water to blender and process until completely smooth.

5 In a large bowl, toss cooked pasta and cheese sauce until completely coated. Spread mixture into a 9 × 12-inch casserole dish, sprinkle with bread crumbs, and dust with paprika. Bake for 30 minutes, or until cheese sauce is bubbling and the bread crumbs are golden brown.

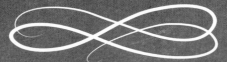

Vegan ≠ Ugly Plastic Shoes

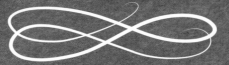

Day 10

*It's true that some vegan shoes are ugly, but so are some leather shoes. Vegan fashion—especially **leather alternatives—is one of the hottest** (and most sustainable) fashion statements out there.*

If you want

to be fashionable—but not fashionably late—then you should probably go vegan immediately. Top luxury brands are ditching animal products in favor of sustainable and chic cruelty-free ones. High-end fashion designers Diane von Fürstenberg and Ralph Lauren—along with 340 other companies—banned mohair, a silklike fabric made from the Angora goat. Fur, another unnecessary and hideously cruel product, has also been ousted by top-tier luxury designers, including Coach, which did so because they said it's "the right thing to do." Suffice it to say, vegan fashion is no longer equated with oversize hemp sacks that vaguely emit the scent of patchouli and moral superiority.

Veganism even has its own fashion week. Debuting in 2018 in Los Angeles, the goal of the game-changing Vegan Fashion Week is to end animal exploitation in all forms by elevating vegan visionaries and educating enthusiasts about the ethical, social, and environmental issues surrounding the use of animals in the industry. The event—which caused ripples throughout the fashion industry and was covered in mainstream media outlets around the world—is positioned to be replicable and scalable in fashion-forward cities globally, in hopes that the more standard fashion week eventually pivots to no longer include the use of animals at all.

Backing this booming industry are such iconic designers as Stella McCartney. In addition to creating revolutionary vegan products, including a vegan leather line of Stan Smith sneakers and an upcoming line of vegan silk, McCartney recently partnered with the United Nations to create a new fashion industry charter for climate action to help fashion companies embrace sustainable and ethical practices. The full charter included sixteen commitments that set a path for collective action to reduce the industry's environmentally damaging effects—such as waste, pollution, deforestation, toxins in manufacturing, and carbon-fueled supply chains. A true ethical pioneer, McCartney created her own fashion label around principles of sustainable and ethical consumption practices. Her best-selling bag, the Falabella, is made from polyester and recycled nylon.

To say it's about time for a colossal, industry-wide shift away from exploitation and toward compassion and sustainability is a gross understatement. Animals used for leather, fur, wool, and silk are horrifically and unnecessarily tortured. For that kind of cruel behavior to be considered standard—all in the name of so-called beauty—is an example of humanity pretty much breaking. The majority of leather comes from developing countries, such as China, Brazil, and India, where animal welfare laws either don't exist or aren't enforced. Stateside, many of the millions of cows and other animals who are killed for their skin are part of the horrific factory farming industry, routinely enduring castration, branding, and tail-docking—without any painkillers. Once at slaughterhouses, it is routine for these individuals to have their throat cut; some are skinned and dismembered while still conscious.

This is tough stuff to wrap your head around, especially when bounteous alternative leather products are high-fashion, highly accessible, and—unlike the environmentally draining process of leather production—actually kind to the planet. At the first Vegan Fashion Week, which attracted top designers, including Dr. Martens and Matea Benedetti, leather analogues were made from the likes of cork (you just skin the bark off the tree, same as you would a breathing animal), pineapple (specifically Piñatex, made from a pineapple leaf), and apple industry waste (an apple a day keeps the animal-skinners away). There's also current development of leathers made from oranges and even coffee grounds (and no, this is not the brunch chapter).

Of course, another industry ripe with horrific cruelty is fur—and some cities, especially in California, are even banning the sale (and sometimes the sale *and* production) of it. These include West Hollywood, Berkeley, Los Angeles, and San Francisco. Across the country in fashion mecca New York City, pending legislation has been introduced which, if passed, would follow suit, banning the sale of cruelly begotten animal skins.

More and more designers are getting the memo that there's nothing even remotely beautiful about torturing animals for their skins or body parts (not to mention, Neanderthal style has been out of fashion since they lost the evolutionary battle to Homo sapiens). A growing number of fashion brands—including Michael Kors, Gucci, Armani, and BCBG—have also agreed to remove fur from their collections.

The reason for these bans is because the production of fur is, to put it mildly, an abomination. Animals on fur farms (including beavers, chinchillas, dogs, cats, foxes, rabbits, raccoons, seals, and bears) spend their days and nights confined in dirty wire cages, with their short and miserable life routinely ended by way of electrocution (vaginal or anal), suffocation, gassing, or poisoning. More than 50 percent of fur in the United States comes from China, and since Chinese fur is often mislabeled, there's no way of knowing which species of animal you're wearing. Many US consumers are horrified to learn that their fur came from a dog or cat, but wouldn't scoff if it had come from a rabbit or beaver—both of whom are extremely social animals who, like dogs and cats, value their family and friends.

This is all a bit crazy, right? Do you need to cuddle your dog? Because we can wait.

Rest assured that like any other industry that relies on exploitation for profit, there are other ways. Do be suspicious of faux fur, however. Although on the plus side, the demand for faux fur has increased over the past ten years, this societal awakening has also resulted in a surplus of real fur. As a result, several big companies, including Barney's, Dillard's, and Neiman Marcus, have sold animal fur labeled as faux. Yes, you read that correctly.

There are, however, vegan faux fur companies you can indeed trust, as they value ethics as highly as they value fashion. These include Unreal Fur, Helen Moore, Donna Salyers' Fabulous Furs, AdelaQueen, LaSeine&Moi, Jakke, FURious Fur, PAWJ, James&Co, Shrimps, Pelush, SpiritHoods, Only Me, Charly Calder, and Apparis. Beyond wearing faux furs that are proven to be ethically created, there are current innovations under way to produce 3D-printed fur alternatives, which would be extremely eco-friendly (more so than some fur alternatives).

Vegan fashion is available from head to toe, literally. At one time, vegans had to rely on cheap shoe stores for style—such as the now defunct Payless (RIP, Payless!)—nowadays, sustainable and gorgeous footwear is easy to come by for those who don't use leather or animal products. You could, of course, still find plenty of leather-free shoes at such places as H&M, Forever 21, or Target—or by scouting around at many thrift stores, including Crossroads Trading Company, Goodwill, or Buffalo Exchange (of course, buying secondhand is also a really solid choice you can make for the planet, and you can find some supercute things). But there are also intentionally vegan lines that are both great to support and are regularly seen on runways, and these include Brave-GentleMan, Cri de Coeur, Veerah, and Matt & Nat.

There is simply no reason to wear animal skins, which is evident when you look around at some of these vegan designers that are keeping things eco-friendly, nonviolent, and simply gorgeous. Leather is a by-product of the meat and dairy industries, and over a hundred million animals are slaughtered each year for their fur. Whether the individual whose skin is being torn from them is a cow (which is most common), or someone more seemingly exotic, such as an alligator, ostrich, or snake, leather production of all kinds is an intensive, laborious process that involves tanning. Tanning uses large amounts of formaldehyde, chrome, cyanide, and arsenic (ARSENIC!). These are all harmful chemicals that not only damage the planet, but also the workers whose job is to handle them . . . all so that we can have a leather

Pleather Principle

With today's luxe-looking leather facsimiles, there's just no excuse for wearing dead animals on your feet, legs, or back. No animals were harmed to make these textiles that have their roots (literally) in nature. Check out the surprise sources behind your next new pair of shoes.

APPLE

The original fruit is so much more versatile than even Eve could have imagined. Besides cold-pressed juices and pie, apples—and, more specifically, their peels—are being transformed by several European manufacturers into fiber that's strong, breathable, and, of course, 100-percent vegan.

PINEAPPLE

Former leather-industry pro Carmen Hijosa began looking for animal-hide alternatives after learning about leather's negative environmental impact, and found what she was searching for in the spiky leaves of the *Ananas comosus* plant (or pineapple, for short). Today, Piñatex is transformed into shoes, bags, and swank fabrics for interior design.

clutch. Assuming the leather is coming from a cow, the process of taking her skin happens after she's already been impregnated and milked at a dairy operation until she is considered "spent" and turned into low-grade beef. It's all part of the same cycle and system; you can't have one without the other.

The cringe-worthy injustices of leather production are not unlike wool production, which relies on painful practices for sheep, including chopping off the ends of tails, castration if he's a boy, and shearing that regularly leaves the sheep cut and bleeding. Merino sheep—who of course produce merino wool—have naturally folded skin, and more skin means more area to grow wool. But this extra skin becomes a breeding ground for flies, so much so that in New Zealand, 2.3 million adult and baby sheep each year are eaten alive by maggots—it's called "flystrike" and is about as fun as it sounds.

All of this information can definitely be overwhelming. Similarly to learning about the cruelty inherent in factory farming, this is the stuff that makes us question everything at the same time as making us want to eat pint after pint of vegan ice cream (if you're gonna, you might as well go for Peanut Butter

MUSHROOMS

Want to be the "fun guy" at the next office shindig? Wear your mushroom-leather cap and get the party started! This pliable, suedelike material breathes like cotton and has natural antibacterial properties that make it particularly well suited to shoes. Who'll be the first to transform it into footwear? Birkenstocks is a shoo-in.

CORK

In Portugal, the epicenter of the cork industry, the bark of the *Quercus suber* tree is sustainably harvested every nine years to create a lightweight, stain-resistant material that's transformed into bags, shoes, and even ultradurable flooring. Eco-conscious designers love its versatility, and the fact that the trees require no pesticides, pruning, or irrigation to grow.

LAB-GROWN

When is leather considered to be a fabric suitable for conscious consumers? Some say when it's made in a laboratory from a few jellyfish cells. Geltor was among the first high-tech companies to develop cruelty-free cultured leather and bring it to market.

Half-Baked from Ben & Jerry's). Not to oversimplify, but for now, just breathe (in between bites), and feel empowered knowing that in this world where we seemingly have so little power over so many things, we can actually control where we put our money. Rest assured that in this inexplicably oppressive system, we can still vote with our dollars—and that wields a lot more power than you might realize.

Rome wasn't built in a day, and neither was a vegan's leather-free shoe collection. You don't have to throw away all of the animal products in your fridge and closet. And though that might be the right way forward for a few people, the truth is, most people who go vegan hold onto their leather belts or shoes for a while, slowly over time replacing them with vegan versions. Be kind to yourself just as you want to be kind to animals (would it be too cheesy to remind you that you're an animal, too?), and don't feel the need to right your wrongs of yesterday immediately—just focus on how to live in ethical alignment with your values as you move forward from here. Thankfully, there's no better way to turn heads than when rocking cruelty-free clothing. Ethics *and* fashion? Oh my god, you're such a catch.

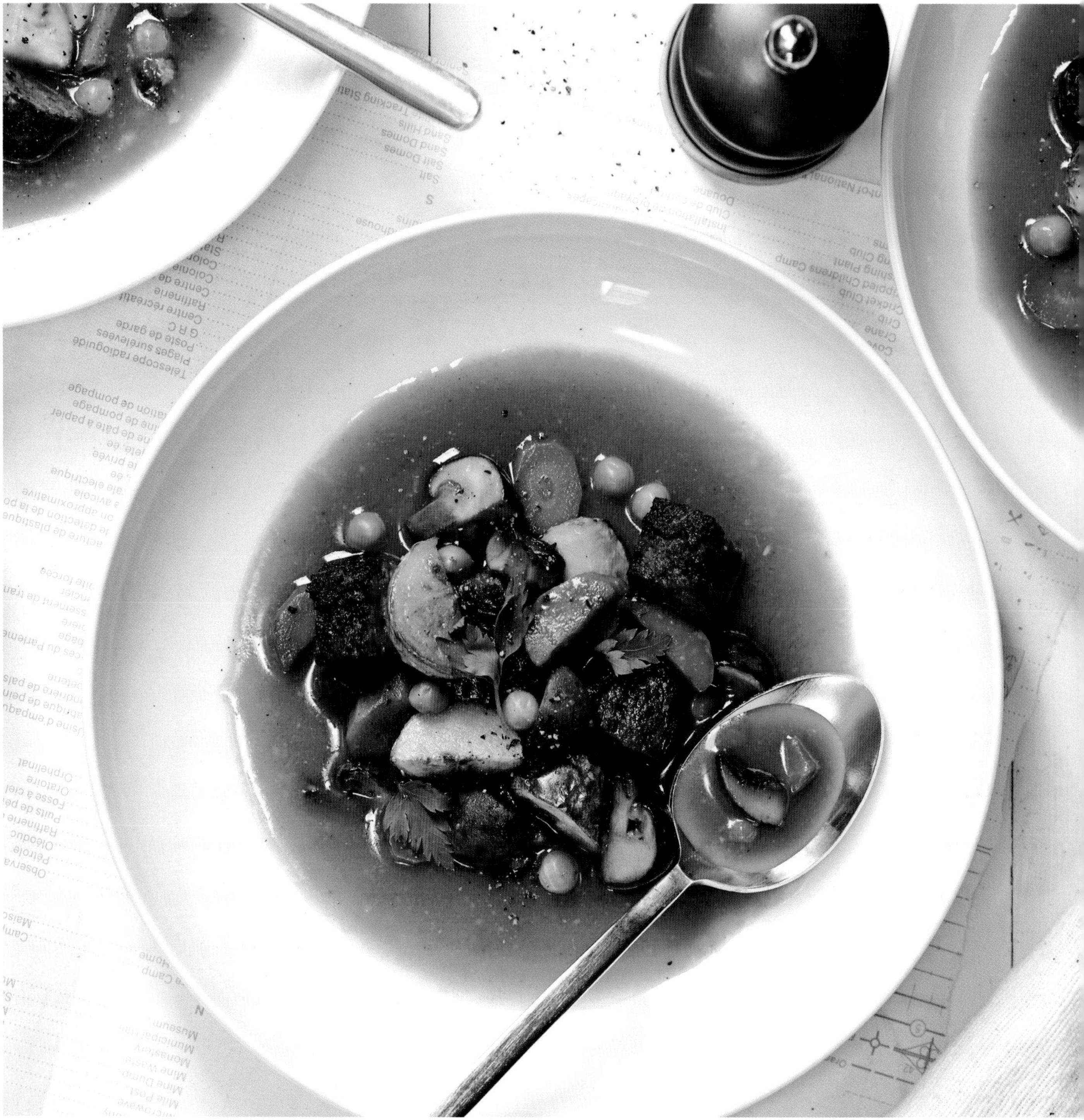

Boeuf Bourguignon

Turn heads with this stunning vegan remake of a classic French stew featuring garlicky vegan beef bathed in a red wine reduction.

Seitan:

3 cups quartered cremini mushrooms
3 tablespoons soy sauce
1 cup vegetable stock
⅓ cup red wine
3 garlic cloves
2 cups vital wheat gluten
1 tablespoon vegetable oil

Red wine sauce:

¼ cup water
3 cups diced onion
2 cups diced celery
2 cups diced carrot
6 ripe tomatoes, chopped
3 cups red wine
1 garlic bulb, cloves separated, peeled, and sliced

12 dried shiitake mushrooms
1 cup sliced cremini mushrooms
¼ cup soy sauce
3 tablespoons medium miso
1 teaspoon dried rosemary
1 teaspoon dried thyme
7½ cups vegetable stock, plus more as needed

Bourguignon:

2½ cups chopped carrot
5 cups halved cremini mushrooms
2½ cups halved baby potatoes
2 cups small green peas
¼ teaspoon salt
¼ teaspoon black pepper
¼ cup vegetable oil
⅔ cup all-purpose flour
½ cup chopped fresh parsley

❶ **Prepare the seitan:** In a food processor, add mushrooms, soy sauce, vegetable stock, red wine, and garlic. Process until combined. Add wheat gluten and process for about 30 seconds, until a soft dough is formed.

❷ Divide dough into five portions and form each into a patty about ½ inch thick. In a skillet over medium heat, heat oil and cook each patty, flipping until browned on both sides.

❸ **Prepare the red wine sauce:** In a large pot or Dutch oven over medium heat, add water and sauté onion, celery, and carrot until tender. Add tomatoes, wine, garlic, shiitake and cremini mushrooms, soy sauce, miso, rosemary, and thyme and bring to a boil. Add vegetable stock and sautéed seitan and bring to a boil again. Cover, lower heat to low, and simmer for 1 hour or longer to concentrate. Add more vegetable stock if flavor is too strong or boil down longer for stronger flavor and thicker sauce.

4 Using tongs, remove seitan from pot and set aside on a plate. Set a colander over a large bowl and pour sauce mixture through to strain vegetables, pressing out as much liquid as possible to yield about 6 cups strained sauce (add additional stock, if needed).

5 **Prepare the bourguignon:** Preheat oven to 425°F. On a baking sheet, arrange carrot, mushrooms, potato, and peas in a single layer, season with salt and pepper, and roast in oven for 25 minutes, or until tender.

6 In a large pot over low heat, heat vegetable oil. Add flour and cook, stirring, for several minutes to make a roux. Add strained sauce and whisk well to incorporate. Cook, stirring with a wooden spoon, until thickened.

7 Chop seitan into 1½-inch chunks and add to sauce along with roasted vegetables. Simmer for 10 minutes, sprinkle with parsley, and serve warm.

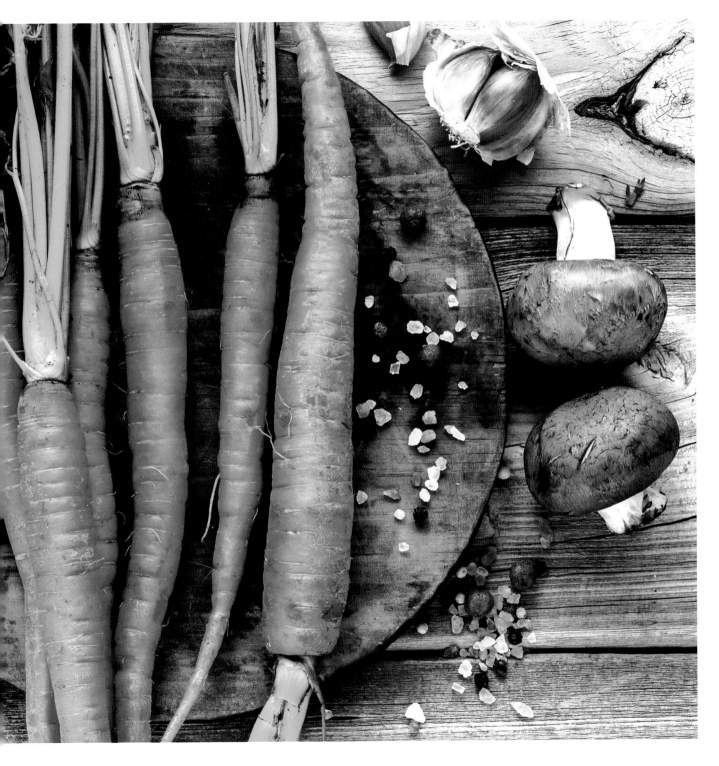

Let Us
Eat Cake!

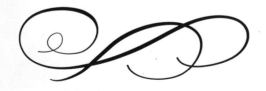

Day 11

*Veganism does not mean deprivation. **Vegans can have their cake** (and doughnuts and pie and brownies) and eat it, too.*

There are

many areas in which vegans excel, but perhaps none as masterfully as dessert. Although we're not sure exactly how many vegan dessert cookbooks exist, our guess would be thousands. That's because there are as many vegan desserts to write about as there are nonvegan ones. And the ease of simple swaps makes plant-based baking a no-brainer. We get to use egg replacers instead of eggs (which might mean a commercial egg replacer, flax or chia seeds, applesauce, mashed banana, silken tofu, arrowroot powder, vinegar and baking soda, dairy-free yogurt, agar-agar, soy lecithin, or aquafaba—otherwise known as the magical liquid in a can of chickpeas); vegan butter instead of dairy-based butter (such as Miyoko's, Earth Balance, or I Can't Believe It's Not Butter's vegan line); and plant-based milk instead of cows' milk (you've got your soy, almond, cashew,

macadamia, peanut, oat, flax, hemp, rice, and on and on). The rest of the ingredients in baking are pretty much the same as the nonvegan recipes, and if you don't happen to have one of those thousands of vegan cookbooks, you can easily swap in vegan stand-ins when using your more generic cookbook. Any food can be pivoted to be vegan—but in baking, it's especially easy.

Many vegans report that when they finally ditch animal products, they discover a whole array of rich tastes and new cuisines that they had never known about before. Veganism can indeed open up a whole plethora of new layers of flavor that will ensure your taste buds will be intensely satisfied. Dessert is no exception. On the contrary, the possibilities of taking a standard, non-vegan dessert and elevating it to fully plant-based are limitless, with the added benefit that since there is no egg in a vegan dessert, you can safely devour all the batter you want without having to worry about *E. coli*. Veganism for the win.

If you're a level one vegan and are brand new to the scene (or if you're trying out plant-based living but it's too soon for you to assign yourself a label), do note that plenty of commercially available desserts are vegan. These include original Oreos, Jell-O pudding mix (add nondairy milk), Hershey's chocolate syrup, Pillsbury crescent rolls, unfrosted Pop-Tarts (the strawberry, blueberry, and sugar-cinnamon varieties), and Teddy Grahams. Even the little Biscoff cookie that is now regularly served on many US flights is vegan, so you can dip it into your terrible black coffee during your cross-country trip and dream about the creamy soy latte you'll enjoy the second you land.

If you're a level five vegan—or someone who wishes to know about the nuanced ins-and-outs of veganism—you might want to learn about the problems in many commercially available sugars (including in those products listed above). Do keep in mind that veganism is about not letting the perfect be the enemy of the good, and there's a lot of value in mainstream companies, such as Nabisco, having superpopular products that don't include animal ingredients, and that should be celebrated and supported—particularly when you're talking about working within highly oppressive systems to ensure that plant-based products exist. Even vegans who choose not to eat Oreos think it's pretty great that Oreos don't include animal products.

That said, here's the problem with sugar, Sugar: there are two sources from which sugar comes from—sugarcane and sugar beets, and in the United States, they are used about equally. But many refined sugars made from sugarcane are filtered through bone char, which is widely used as a decolorizing filter (to give it that bright white color). The bones originate from cows in countries that include Argentina, India, Pakistan, and Afghanistan (notably, they can't come from the United States because the FDA prohibits using bones from the meat industry due to health concerns, so we import them and let others do the dirty work for us), are then sold to traders, and those traders sell them to the US sugar industry. Sugar that is filtered through bones takes the shape of products including (but not limited to) brown sugar and powdered sugar, but supermarket brands get their sugar from many different refineries—so one cannot know for sure if the sugar was filtered with bones (with the exception of organic sugar, which is *not* filtered through bone char). Beet sugar is never processed with bone char, since it does not need the same decolorization. Instead, the beets' juice is removed through a diffuser, and then that juice is crystalized after it is mixed with additives. Bone char: it's what's for dinner.

In her book *Sweet + Salty: The Art of Vegan Chocolates, Truffles, Caramels, and More*, ethical chocolatier and author Lagusta Yearwood explains how the sugar industry is fraught with problems, and the importance of being a conscious consumer. She says, "Unlike chocolate, no one really seems to care about how sugar gets to us. Spoiler: it's not pretty. Land grabs by massive sugar conglomerates that displace indigenous people, deforest and destroy already fragile ecosystems, and threaten habitat loss; excessive fertilizer usage that results in poisoned water and soils; working conditions that include child labor, massive inhumanities, and yep, forced labor." This searing reality is anything but sweet, and Yearwood goes on to explain how "Sugar is one of the most sickeningly political agricultural products we come into daily contact with—and has been for hundreds of years."

You could indeed make yourself crazy thinking about all of the sideline issues—such as sugar sourcing and filtering agents—and the last thing you should feel you need to do when trying vegan is to throw your hands in the air and say, "I give up!" Even plenty of longtime vegans don't pay close attention to the processing of such foods as sugar; as long as there is no meat, milk, and eggs included as actual ingredients, many vegans are fine. This is especially true when you are dining out and you order, for example, the slice of vegan cake on the menu. There's a lot of value in ordering it and showing the eatery that there's a demand for vegan desserts, so it's not usually a top priority to inquire about the sourcing of their sugar. But when you're buying sugar at the store, you might take that extra step to make sure that you're supporting brands that are vegan and look for that organic label (brands Florida Crystals, Now Real Food Beet Sugar,

Rapunzel Organic Whole Cane Sugar, Sugar in the Raw, Trader Joe's, and Wholesome are among those that are all vegan).

Many people who go vegan find a great new hobby in baking, because it's one of the simplest and most satisfying activities. There's also the added benefit of sharing the fruits—or the cupcakes—of your labor. There's no single better way to advocate for animals and the environment than through sharing delicious food, and many new vegans take that concept to new heights, baking delectable goodies for everyone they've ever met in their entire life. Just think, you can be that person who brings better-than-Grandma's banana bread, chocolate chip cookies, and our favorite—Salted Caramel Brownies (lucky for you, the recipe follows!)—to the office.

There are also plenty of store-bought cake and brownie mixes that are vegan, as long as you add your own egg-replacer, dairy-free butter, and plant-based milk. These include mixes (check the labels!) from Duncan Hines, Simple Mills, Miss Jones Baking Co., Food Stirs, Bob's Red Mill, Madhava, It's Wholesome, Kiki's Gluten Free, Pillsbury, and more. So, even if you don't fancy yourself a Betty Crocker, you can fool people into thinking you are. Plus, even though there are plenty of high-end, artisanal vegan desserts, sometimes there's nothing better than a sloppily frosted, slightly leaning cake with messy rainbow sprinkles.

Swap This For That

In baking, there are some very simple swaps you can make to ensure that anything nonvegans can bake, vegans can bake better. Here's how to start.

SWAP OUT COWS' MILK FOR COCONUT MILK

The purpose of milk is to add moisture to a batter. Canned coconut milk naturally contains a significant amount of fat, which provides even more moisture and a silkier mouthfeel than cows' milk. Don't worry—you won't taste the coconut.

SWAP OUT BUTTER FOR VEGAN BUTTER

It's a simple one-to-one swap. Both Melt Organic and Earth Balance make vegan butter in stick form, so you can easily swap these in for your famous (or soon-to-be-famous) cookie, pie dough, and frosting recipes.

SWAP OUT EGG WHITES FOR AQUAFABA

Technically, aquafaba is the brine left over from a can of chickpeas, but we like to call it "vegan magic." Use 3 tablespoons of aquafaba per egg, and add a pinch of cream of tartar to stabilize when whipping into fluffy white peaks. Aquafaba makes perfect meringues and pavlovas, but you can use it in cakes and brownies, too.

SWAP OUT EGGS FOR APPLESAUCE

In most quick breads, muffins, and brownies, use ¼ cup applesauce to replace each egg. The puréed fruit acts as a binder, just as an egg would in these recipes.

SWAP OUT EGGS FOR CIDER VINEGAR AND BAKING SODA

Yes, we've already listed eggs, but eggs do different things in different baked goods. In cakes, you want your batter to rise—applesauce won't do that, but the combo of 1 tablespoon of cider vinegar mixed with 1 teaspoon of baking soda will make your cakes light and airy.

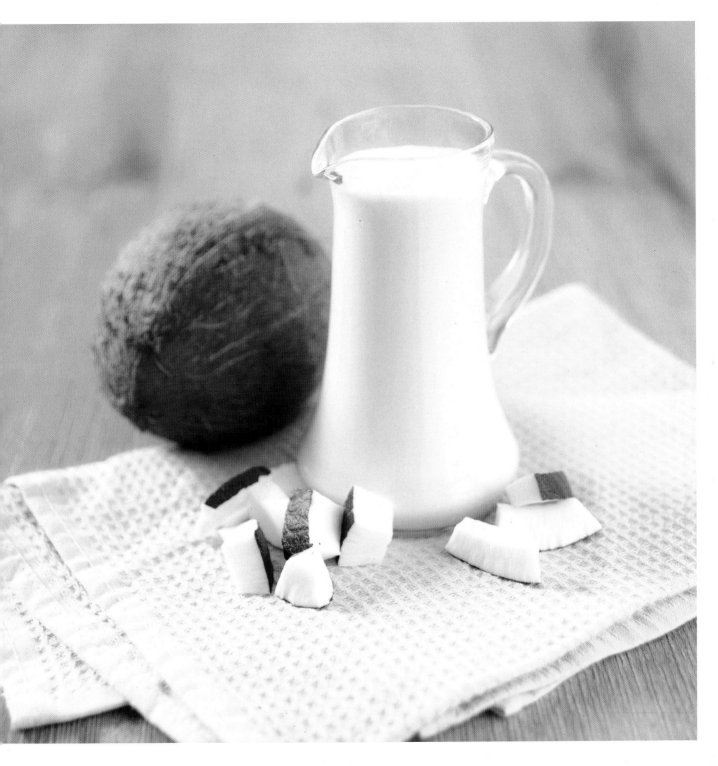

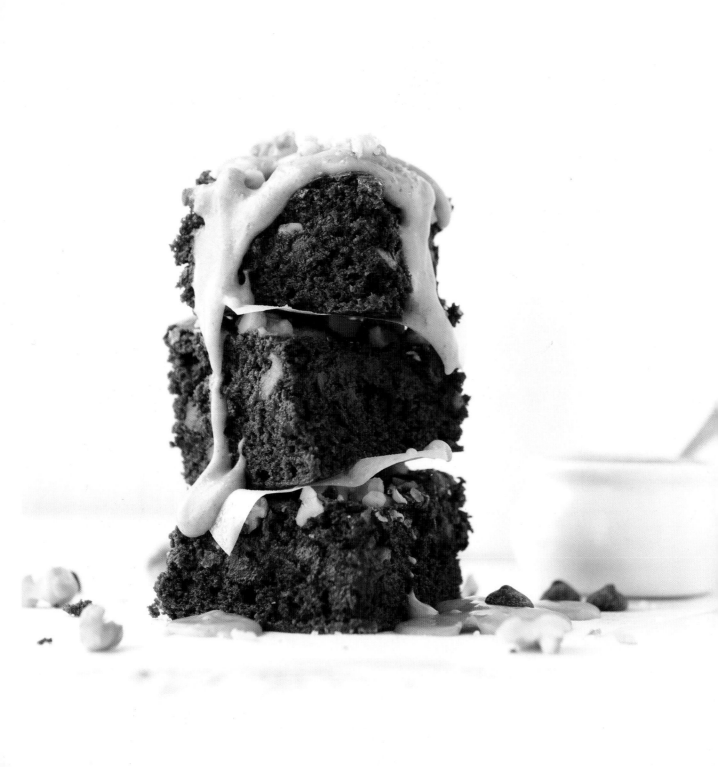

Salted Caramel Brownies

Fudgy, walnut-studded double chocolate brownies topped with a thick, luscious caramel sauce means you're guaranteed to be racing through dinner to get to dessert.

Brownies:

Cooking spray, for pan

2   cups all-purpose flour

⅔   cup unsweetened cocoa powder

2   teaspoons baking powder

½   teaspoon salt

1   cup unsweetened vegan milk

1   cup granulated sugar

⅔   cup light brown sugar

½   cup coconut oil, melted

2   tablespoons ground flaxseeds

1   teaspoon pure vanilla extract

¼   cup vegan chocolate chunks

½   cup chopped walnuts

Salted date caramel:

1   cup pitted dates

1   cup full-fat canned coconut milk

¼   teaspoon salt

⅛   teaspoon coarse sea salt, for garnish

1 **Prepare the brownies:** Preheat oven to 350°F. Line an 8-inch square baking dish with parchment paper, extending the paper over two opposite sides for easy lifting, and lightly coat with cooking spray.

2 Into a large bowl, sift flour, cocoa, baking powder, and salt. In a small bowl, whisk together milk, granulated sugar, brown sugar, coconut oil, flaxseeds, and vanilla. Add wet mixture to dry and stir until just combined. Fold in chocolate chunks and ¼ cup of walnuts into batter.

3 Pour batter into prepared baking dish. Sprinkle with remaining ¼ cup of walnuts. Bake for 30 to 35 minutes, or until the top has risen and does not jiggle. Remove from oven and place baking dish on a wire rack to cool for 1 hour.

4 **Prepare the salted date caramel:** Soak dates in warm water for 10 minutes if not already soft. Drain, reserving water. In a blender, combine dates, coconut milk, and salt and blend until very smooth. If necessary, add reserved date water 1 teaspoon at a time and blend mixture until warm.

5 Once brownies have cooled, carefully lift out of baking dish by pulling up parchment paper. Slice into sixteen squares, drizzle with salted date caramel, and lightly sprinkle with coarse sea salt. Serve immediately or refrigerate brownies and caramel separately for up to 1 week.

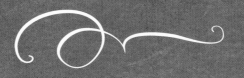

Eyeshadow Is for Humans, Not Bunnies

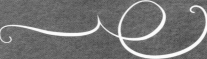

Day 12

Cosmetic animal testing is cruel and unnecessary, which is why it's on the outs. But **cruelty-free, vegan makeup is available everywhere**, *including your local drugstore.*

Although it's

not terribly uncommon for some (not-yet-enlightened) people to still have hang-ups about the word *vegan*, you'd be hard-pressed to find anyone who would argue that animal testing for cosmetics is okay. The cognitive dissonance around somehow normalizing this practice—a societal blind spot that's carried out by continuing to patronize companies that rely on painful practices, such as forcing animals to ingest a substance like shampoo until they die, so as to find out how much it takes to kill them—is inexplicable. Yet we do it, because that's how deeply entrenched media and marketing schemes are. These products promise flawless skin, perfectly blushed cheeks, and impeccable eyebrows.

How is it possible that these same products that are touted in magazine ads and TV commercials as beautifying are, at their root, promoting heartless cruelty to caged animals? No, this can't be right. Surely there are laws that protect animals from undergoing needless tests that blind rabbits. Maybe tests like that happen overseas where there are fewer regulations . . . but here? Nah. Those images of a small animal whose eyes are permanently shut due to infection from hair dye being poured into them to see whether it is safe for humans—an entirely different species whose body reacts differently to stimuli anyway—could not *possibly* be intentional. She must have been blind from birth. Maybe she accidentally walked into a sharp object and caused it herself. Or maybe . . . it's Maybelline.

Animal testing. It's one of those things that most of us don't ever wrap our heads around, especially when we find ourselves at the 24-hour Rite Aid drugstore searching for emergency hair dye because our roommate's peroxide we found under the sink didn't quite have the beach-blonde effect we had hoped it would in our impulsive quest of a late-night makeover. So, we run into the store and grab the first thing we see, not even giving any thought to how that product came to be.

This is unfortunate, because that same drugstore that carries those cruel products also carries cruelty-free, vegan selections, products whose companies went a different route entirely—doing what it took to get a beauty product on the market that never once relied on the torture of animals to make us pretty. So, the question looms: if some companies can figure out how to create products without the use of animals, why don't all of them?

If you feel like it, you can repeat out loud the big takeaway from this book right now: that there's a (fabulous) vegan version of everything, beauty products included. This is really good news; you don't need to sacrifice your ethics to look good. Now that you know there are ethical ways forward (and you don't even have to go out of your way to find special stores, since all stores carry cruelty-free cosmetics— you just need to know what to look for), let's unpack what's really going on with animal testing.

In the United States alone, more than 800,000 animals used in labs are used to test cosmetics, chemicals, and pharmaceuticals each year (this doesn't include mice, rats, or fish—adding that would push that number up to the millions). The cost to do so? $12 billion—though it could be much higher when considering all the products tested on animals—and a whole lot of egregious cruelty for no reason—especially considering the cruelty-free alternatives that are literally within our reach.

First things first: the entire basis of animal testing is based on a flawed premise, which is that nonhuman animal bodies undergoing chemical reactions will respond the same way as human bodies. This is, gravely, not true. Animal testing for cosmetics is brutish and savage, initially instituted in order to supposedly test the side effects and efficacy of products. The Draize test—devised in 1944—was originally used for cosmetics testing and involved applying a substance to an awake, restrained animal's eyeballs or skin and leaving the substance there for up to two weeks to monitor such reactions as hemorrhaging and blindness. Nearly all animals in tests are killed afterward; very occasionally, animals may be reused, but most of the time, they are murdered and dissected.

One of the most tragic parts of this grossly inhumane test is the fact that it's useless, due to the difference between humans' eyes and rabbits', for example, as well as the subjective nature of a visual evaluation. In some cases, rabbits' eyelids are clipped so that they are forced to remain open during the testing; the little bodies are placed in restraining devices so they can't move, as oftentimes their eyes are left bleeding and ulcerated due to the chemicals in them. Rabbits don't produce tears as we do, so they can't wash the chemicals out of their eyes. The Draize test for skin irritancy involves the test substance being applied to animals' skin, which is then abraded—meaning, many layers of skin are removed with sticky tape.

(Hang in there. We're almost done.)

Animals used in labs are also regularly force-fed—a tube is inserted into their esophagus and stomach—to determine how much of a substance they are able to tolerate. This process, which almost always kills them, is excruciating, leading to tumors and gene mutations.

For the most part, cosmetics are not actually required to undergo animal testing in the United States, but there are exceptions—such as some anti-bacterial soaps, sunscreens, and dandruff shampoos. But companies are still responsible for making sure that their ingredients and finished products are safe prior to that product coming to market. These days, many companies actually don't have a need to test because their formulas are considered "generally recognized as safe," but some companies continue to conduct animal testing as an added layer of legal protection, should there one day be a lawsuit due to a product hurting a human. Companies that market or manufacture overseas (such as China) may also be required to submit these products for testing; however, an increasing amount of countries world-wide have passed laws banning cosmetics testing on animals.

Stateside, legislation banning animal testing is also on the up and up. In 2018, California passed the California Cruelty-Free Cosmetics Act. This landmark act bans the sale of animal-tested beauty products within the state and keeps all noncompliant items off the shelves, making California the first state in the United States to enact such legislation. Let's think about this: if the land of Hollywood and glamour can pull off cruelty-free cosmetics, any state can.

Well ahead of the United States is the European Union, which—back in 2013—banned cosmetic animal testing entirely. In order to sell within the EU, companies simply had to develop cruelty-free formulas. Within the subsequent five years, India, Israel, Turkey, Switzerland, Guatemala, Taiwan, and Norway all issued similar bans.

So, what are the alternatives to cruel and inhumane animal testing for cosmetics? In-vitro testing—such as cultivating three-dimensional human skin cells, and computer modeling—are ethical innovations that frequently cost less to implement, have better accuracy, and do not rely on the exploitation of any animal. Even the National Institutes of Health and the US Department of Defense have funded revolutionary organs-on-chips toxicology models.

Ethical solutions that are already available have proven to be more cost-effective and accurate than the antiquated and barbaric animal testing practices. This includes a method known as RASAR (read-across structure activity relationships), which provides companies access to a sharable database of ten thousand common toxic chemicals. There's not only hope in this shared database, but also in the shared perspective that when it comes to animal testing for cosmetics, vegans are not the only ones who think it's barbaric. Poll after poll proves that people don't want their cosmetics with a side of bunny blindness, and as more companies are getting that memo—and understanding that there are countless ethical alternatives that are way more cost-effective and productive than truly horrifying practices involving animals—the country and the world are moving toward creating products that reflect our values.

Keep in mind that unpacking the confusing language of beauty product labeling can sometimes be less straightforward than it should. Labels can be misleading, since in the beauty business, "cruelty-free" is defined as not being tested on animals, but "vegan" means made entirely from plant-based products. What this means is that products labeled "cruelty-free" might actually contain animal-derived ingredients (such as goat milk or bee pollen), whereas some vegan products might have undergone animal testing.

This can be crazy-making, but there are ways around it, and you can ensure that your beauty products are both vegan *and* cruelty-free. The Coalition for Consumer Information on Cosmetics keeps more than a thousand companies documented by certifying brands through its Leaping Bunny program. A thorough list of cruelty-free and vegan companies—categorized by cosmetics, animal care, household items, personal care, and others—can be found on Leaping Bunny's website (leapingbunny.org).

Beauty doesn't need to hurt. And until we live in a truly cruelty-free world, doing that extra minute of research to make sure the mascara you're about to buy doesn't have a deep, dark backstory is easy and—for those of us who want to live in alignment with our values—completely necessary. Make the choice to be humane, because, as L'Oréal would say, "you're worth it." So are the animals.

The Future of Testing

Findings show that animal experiments have limited accuracy in predicting human responses, leaving a massive and dangerous margin for error. Fortunately, cutting-edge technologies are being developed to provide much higher accuracy with zero animal suffering.

COMPUTER MODELING

Sophisticated computer models of everything from the brain to the musculoskeletal system can yield reliable results in medical testing using current medical data. What's more, the accuracy of these models can even be improved upon as more advancements are made and information is gained.

ORGANS-ON-CHIPS

Developed by Harvard University's Wyss Institute, this breakthrough technology uses thumb drive–sized, clear microchips embedded with human cells that can accurately model the functions of a number of human organs, including the liver, the lungs, and even the female reproductive system.

SKIN SAMPLING

Donated human skin tissue provides invaluable potential in understanding the effects of different chemicals and substances. The infamous Draize skin test that exposes millions of rabbits to horrifying irritants can predict human skin reaction with 60 percent accuracy, whereas donated human skin is up to 86 percent accurate.

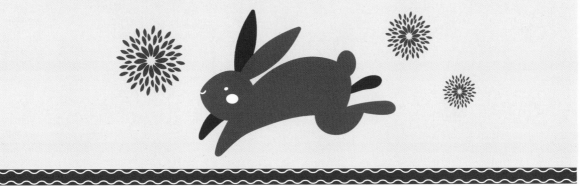

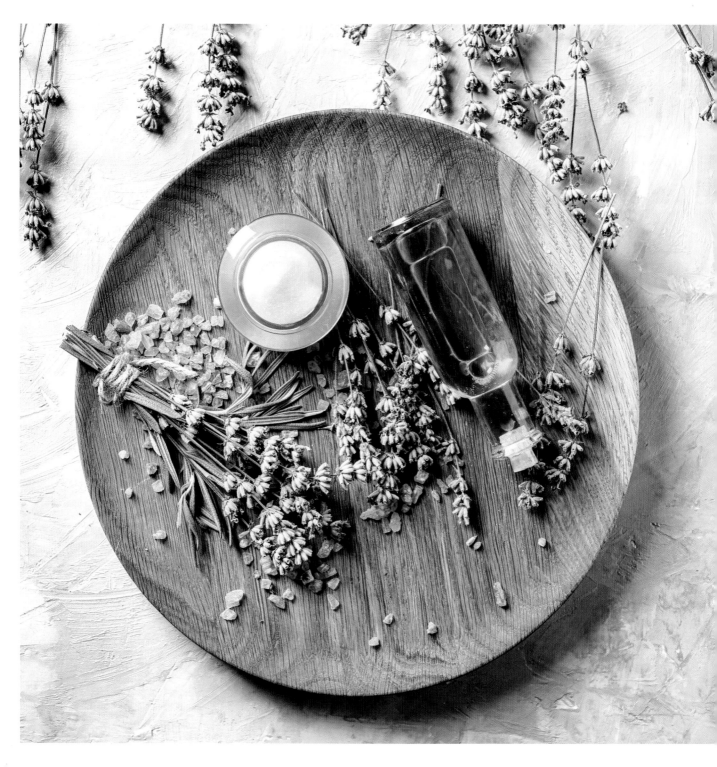

Lavender Sugar Scrub

Antioxidant-rich olive oil provides an emollient base for this easy-to-make scrub. Sugar gently polishes the skin and doesn't break down in the oil the way salt does. Add a few drops of lavender oil for a soothing aromatherapy experience.

1   cup sugar
5 to 10 drops lavender essential oil
½   cup olive oil

In a shallow, wide-mouth jar, combine sugar and lavender essential oil. Pour olive oil over sugar mixture, screw on lid tightly, and shake for 1 minute to blend. To use, moisten face with warm water, then gently massage a teaspoon-size scoop of scrub over your skin, avoiding eye area. Rinse with warm water.

~~~~~~

Peppermint Body Balm

Untoasted extra-virgin sesame oil soothes the skin and offers natural sun protection, while coconut oil gives this creamy balm its structure. Peppermint's invigorating aroma helps lift your mood and make dry feet, hands, and elbows tingle in the best possible way.

¼   cup refined liquid coconut oil
⅛   cup cold-pressed sesame oil
5 to 10 drops peppermint essential oil

In a small jar, combine all ingredients. Screw on lid tightly and shake for 1 minute to blend. Refrigerate until set, then apply liberally to the body, avoiding face and other sensitive areas.

The Cheese (Non-)Quandary

Day 13

*Every single person who has gone vegan has uttered the sentence "But I could never live without cheese" . . . then realized that **vegan cheese is actually the greatest thing on earth.***

It's a wonder

why so many people, when faced with even the most tangential mention of veganism, react so strongly and emotionally—stating that they could "never give up cheese!" If we had a slice of dairy-free provolone for every time someone said that, we could open a vegan cheese factory.

But Miyoko Schinner beat us to making that factory, revolutionizing vegan cheese—and thus, veganism—forever. Her production plant in Northern California is where her artisanal food company, Miyoko's Creamery, creates its myriad umami-rich concoctions. These include a mouthwatering collection of gourmet cheese wheels, luscious cream cheese, and pub-style spreadable cheese perfect for pretzels. She even makes vegan butter. And the rich, flavorful, layered taste profile is seriously nuts. No,

seriously: it's nuts! It's literally made out of cashews (fear not, allergy-sufferers, because an oat-based butter has already hit the shelves).

And it's not just Schinner who's reinventing the cheese wheel. Once you bite into a piece of pizza made with meltable Mozzarella Shreds from Daiya Foods—or a slice of cheese from one of the other dozens of plant-based companies also changing the food game, such as Treeline, Kite Hill, Violife, Field Roast Chao, or Follow Your Heart—you will understand that the hype is real. Although, admittedly, the advent of vegan cheese had, in its earlier days, a margin of error, these days, the product has largely been perfected. This is thanks to innovative chefs and food entrepreneurs who have fine-tuned the nondairy cheese pull—hitting just the right tasty "funk" or getting the gooey, melty texture exactly spot-on—ensuring that cows' milk can be saved for the baby cows it was made for.

Cheese, of course, comes from a lactating cow (which also means you're actually ingesting that cow's estrogen—the female sex hormone). She has to either be pregnant or have just given birth, and since the milk she made was for her baby—just as our mothers' milk is made to nourish us—her offspring need to be removed from her so that she can be hooked up to a machine that takes her milk for human consumption instead. Otherwise, her baby would drink the milk, since that's what babies do (the miracle of life and all that).

Mama needs to be repeatedly kept pregnant, and that is the lot of a dairy cow. That means she's inseminated over and over again (which means that on the other end, a steer's semen is forcibly extracted from him); her babies are routinely taken from her (the boys become veal calves—whereby they are fed an iron-deficient diet so that their flesh stays extra supple—and the girls become dairy cows themselves); and then, when she is considered "spent" (no longer able to produce milk at a high volume), she is killed for low-grade beef (low-grade because her body has been so beat up for so long). It's really a horrific process and is made that much sadder by the knowledge that a mother's instinct to love her baby exists across species, so just like humans, cows cry and bellow when their babies are removed from them. It's all very tragic, especially when you consider how unnecessary, environmentally devastating, and truly unhealthful dairy actually is.

By the way, let it be known that cheese is not necessarily a vegetarian product, which is thanks to the *udderly* (sorry not sorry) disgusting product, rennet (or rennin). Although rennet can sometimes be derived from nonanimal sources (though obviously they're all made with animal-derived milk), many cheeses are made with this enzyme, which comes from a calves' stomach lining. The purpose of these enzymes is to help a nursing baby digest mama's milk, but in cheese-making, it's considered a coagulant. After the baby calf (from the veal industry, which as you now know is a by-product of the dairy industry) is slaughtered, his fourth stomach—which contains these enzymes—is removed, dried, cleaned, and then sliced into tiny pieces and placed into an extraction solution, which after several days, will be filtered. *Say "cheese."*

Beyond the difficult-to-digest truth about where cheese comes from, the health problems associated with dairy consumption are substantial. For one, cheese is extremely high in saturated fat and cholesterol—even 2% milk has 0.2 grams of trans fat, a substance the FDA says we should never eat, not even a little bit. But the dairy industry is tricky about this. Foods that contain between 0 and 0.5 grams of trans fat don't have to include it on their nutrition label, so while your gallon of 2% might be labeled as containing 0 grams, don't be fooled. And dairy can be a major player in a variety of health issues, from the merely uncomfortable to the deadly. As one example, it can stimulate unregulated cell growth, increasing one's risk for hormone-dependent cancers, including prostate.

And hold onto your almonds and soybeans, because this next part is really going to make you mad. Dairy production is not only ripe with health, environmental, and animal-rights problems, but it's a perfect example of institutionalized racism. Yep, racism. Although most humans' bodies are unable to process lactose (a whopping 65 percent of the global population), the prevalence is way higher in African, Asian, Hispanic, and Indigenous people. 70 to 75 percent of African Americans are lactose-intolerant—as well as 95 to 98 percent of Asian Americans, 74 percent of Indigenous, and 53 to 58 percent of Hispanic Americans. Whereas among those with Northern European heritage, it's only around 33 to 35 percent (that's because dairy foods were much more common among people with European ancestry—they have not been a part of the culture and cuisines of communities of color, traditionally). The baseless recommendations to include these foods in the dietary guidelines for communities of color can't be justified any more than it can be digested.

An animal-centric diet is creating disproportionate levels of disease among people of color. By encouraging individuals to consume a Western diet, the government (which sets forth USDA dietary guidelines that still puts focus on dairy) is knowingly promoting excess rates of disease in communities of color. To do this deliberately is racism, plain and simple.

Despite the inequities, health consequences, and environmental implications (for every glass of milk you don't drink, you save the water equivalent of more than a thirty-minute shower—and on top of that, 1.2 billion pounds of waste is produced each day by the global dairy cattle population), people still grasp firmly onto their cheese like it's going to love them back. But, we get it; you can never give up cheese. Back to our favorite phrase: there is a high-quality vegan version of everything. Think of what you typically put cheese on and seek out plant-based alternatives. There are seriously so many alternatives. Store-bought, homemade, nut-free, vegan options in restaurants, the list goes on. This is especially true for pizza places; from indie pizzerias to such chains as Pieology, Blaze, and Fresh Brothers, you can enjoy an ooey-gooey slice of pizza without the legal amount of pus allowed in milk (yep, we went there; the average glass of milk in the United States contains a drop of pus. Truth).

You can even find quality vegan cheese that stretches and melts. Tofu feta? Yep, it's a thing. Cashew and nooch-based Parm? Now *that's* addictive, and nobody even needed to die to get that umami-rich flavor blast.

Cheese Craving

There's a vegan cheese for every hankering out there.
Here are just a few of our faves, perfect for any occasion.

SHRED IT

- ☐ **DAIYA:** Cheddar, Mozzarella, Pepperjack, and Classic

- ☐ **FOLLOW YOUR HEART:** Mozzarella, Fiesta Blend, and Cheddar

- ☐ **GOOD PLANET:** Mozzarella, Smoked Mozzarella, Parmesan, and Cheddar

- ☐ **SO DELICIOUS:** Mozzarella, Cheddar Jack, and Cheddar

- ☐ **VIOLIFE:** Original, Mild Cheddar, and Mozzarella

WEDGE IT

- ☐ **DR-COW:** Aged Cashew Nuts, Aged Macadamia Nuts, Aged Cashew & Brazil Nuts, Aged Cashew & Hemp Seeds, Aged Cashew & Dulse Flakes, Aged Cashew & Blue Green Algae, and Aged Cashew & Kale

- ☐ **MIYOKO'S KITCHEN:** High Sierra Rustic Alpine, Aged English Sharp Farmhouse, Aged English Smoked Farmhouse, and Country Style Herbes de Provence

- ☐ **TREELINE:** Classic Aged Nut Cheese and Cracked Pepper Aged Nut Cheese

SLICE IT

- ☐ **FIELD ROAST CHAO SLICES:** Creamy Original, Coconut Herb, and Tomato Cayenne

- ☐ **FOLLOW YOUR HEART:** American Style Slices, Smoked Gouda Style Slices, Medium Cheddar Style Slices, Provolone Style Slices, Pepper Jack Style Slices, and Mozzarella Style Slices

- ☐ **PARMELA CREAMERY:** American Style, Cheddar, and Pepper Jack Style

- ☐ **TOFUTTI:** American and Mozzarella

SCHMEAR IT

- ❑ **DAIYA:** Plain, Strawberry, Garden Vegetable, and Chive & Onion
- ❑ **FOLLOW YOUR HEART:** Original
- ❑ **KITE HILL:** Everything Bagel, Jalapeño, Strawberry, Plain, and Chive
- ❑ **LEAF CUISINE:** Smokey Gouda, Peppery Jack, Ranch, Garlicky Herb, Presto Pesto, and Beet's Treat
- ❑ **WAYFARE FOODS:** Original, Green Olive, Jalapeño, and Onion Chive

CHEESE BOARD IT

- ❑ **PARMELA CREAMERY:** Black Pepper, Kalamata Olive, and Original
- ❑ **TREELINE:** Herb-Garlic Soft French-Style, Scallion Soft French-Style, Chipotle-Serrano Soft French-Style, and Green Peppercorn Soft French-Style

- ❑ **WAYFARE:** Cheddar and Jalapeño and Cheddar

SPRINKLE IT

- ❑ **PARMA!:** Chipotle Cayenne, Garlicky Green, and Parmesan
- ❑ **PARMELA FOODS:** Parmesan Style
- ❑ **THE VEGETARIAN EXPRESS:** Parma Zaan Sprinkles

NACHO IT

- ❑ **SIETE:** Mild Nacho and Spicy Blanco
- ❑ **NACHEEZ:** Medium, Mild, and Spicy
- ❑ **THE HONEST STAND:** Mild Nacho Dip and Spicy Nacho Dip
- ❑ **WAYFARE:** Nacho Cheddar

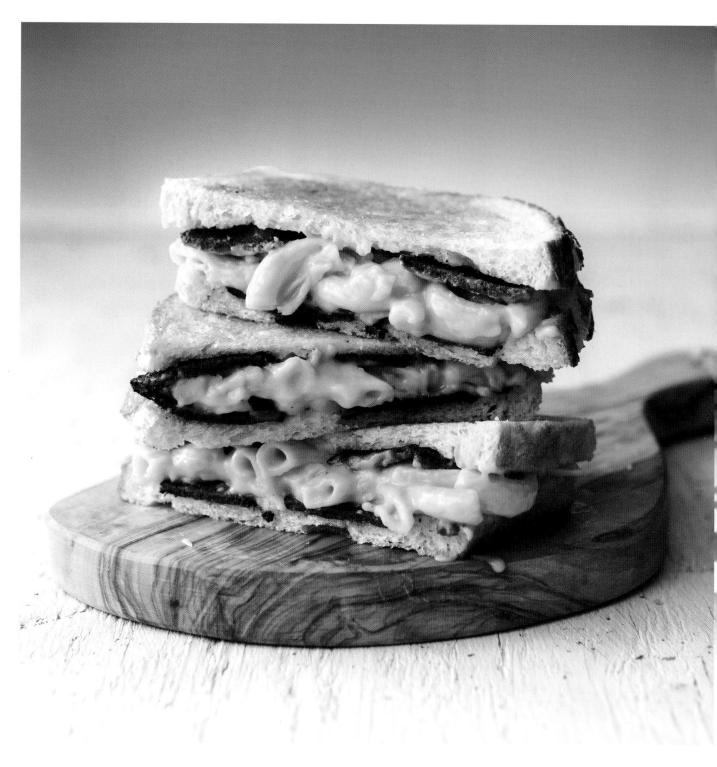

Grilled Bacon Mac & Cheese Sandwiches   Makes 4

What's better than a grilled cheese sandwich? A grilled cheese sandwich filled with bacon and mac & cheese!

Butternut squash mac & cheese:

- ⅔ cup peeled, seeded, and chopped butternut squash
- ½ cup peeled and chopped Yukon Gold potato
- ¼ cup chopped yellow onion
- 1 tablespoon chopped roasted red pepper
- 1 tablespoon olive oil
- 1 garlic clove
- ½ teaspoon cider vinegar
- ½ teaspoon freshly squeezed lemon juice
- ½ teaspoon salt
- 1¼ cups dried elbow pasta
- ¼ cup vegan Cheddar cheese shreds

For assembly:

- 1 tablespoon sunflower oil
- 16 vegan bacon strips
- ¼ cup vegan butter
- 8 slices vegan sourdough bread

1 **Prepare the mac & cheese:** In a medium-size soup pot, combine butternut squash, potato, and onion. Add water to cover, cover with lid, and bring to a boil over medium heat. Boil for 15 minutes, or until fork-tender.

2 Drain water from pot, reserving ¼ cup of liquid. In a blender, combine boiled vegetables, red pepper, oil, garlic, vinegar, lemon juice, and salt and purée until smooth, adding reserved liquid 1 tablespoon at a time to aid with blending.

3 Cook pasta according to package instructions. Drain, return to pot, and stir butternut mixture and Cheddar cheese into pasta until incorporated. Keep warm over low heat.

4 **Prepare the sandwiches:** In a large skillet over medium-high heat, heat oil. Add bacon strips and cook until browned on each side. Remove from skillet, drain on paper towels, and set aside.

5 Butter both sides of each slice of bread. To assemble, lay out four slices of bread and layer each with two strips of bacon, one-quarter of mac & cheese, and two more slices of bacon. Top with remaining four slices of bread and toast sandwiches on a skillet over medium heat until browned. Flip carefully and toast other side. Serve hot.

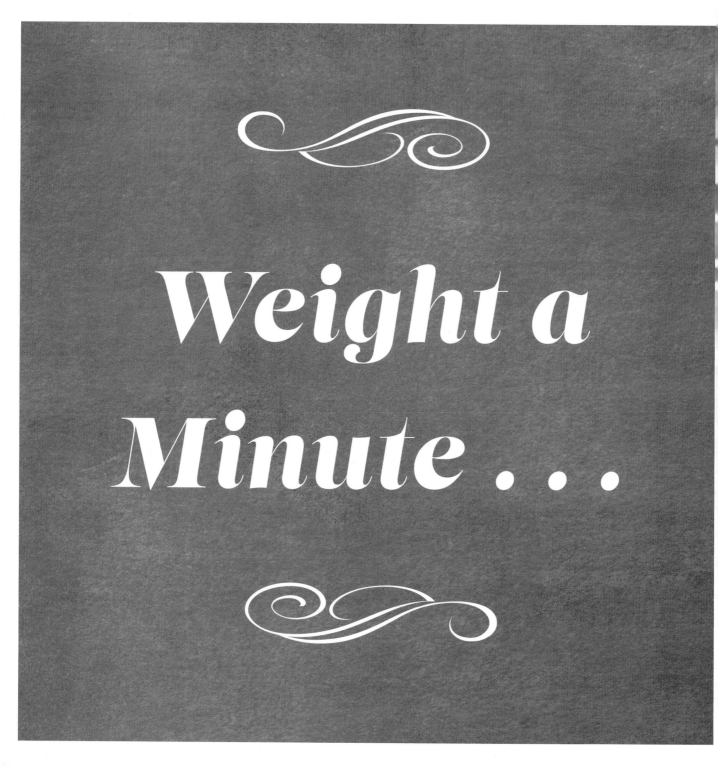

Day 14

Veganism isn't necessarily a weight-loss regimen, but it's superhealthy and can be easily tweaked and personalized **to help you lose (or gain, if you want to) weight.**

For a lot of

vegans, the main impetus for not eating animal products is compassion for animals and the understanding that we can vote with our dollars—which includes boycotting an inherently unethical industry that is also destroying the planet. For many of these people, weight is neither here nor there; it's not even remotely the driving force for their veganism.

A similar—and admittedly odd comparison, but bear with us—is the whole gluten-free craze.

First up, veganism is not the same thing as being gluten-free. Perhaps second to the protein myth, one of the most perplexing (yet not uncommon) things vegans experience is witnessing others' vast confusion between plant-based and gluten-free diets (also, OMG! How is this a thing?). It's like saying that baseball is the same thing as tap-dancing; it doesn't make sense.

Additionally, just as randomly ditching gluten will not by itself result in weight loss—nor is a GF lifestyle first and foremost a weight-loss plan—going vegan isn't synonymous with dieting. The thing about gluten-free diets is that they are completely necessary for those who suffer from celiac disease—otherwise known as an intolerance to gluten—but this serious autoimmune disease affects just 1 percent of the population. Some people have sensitivities, including a nonceliac wheat allergy—but again, restricting your diet for these reasons generally has little to do with weight, or veganism.

How does all of this affect weight? The same way that nonvegan foods affect weight. But when one eats only plants, the decision of whether to lose, maintain, or gain can be a bit more straightforward than when one is on an omnivorous diet, since the animal products are already off the plate. Done and done.

It's time to talk about how to use the foods you consume throughout your day to their optimal benefit to achieve the weight you so desire. Then, we'll focus on celebrating your body, at any size. Remember that vegan diets (with or without gluten, since *they're not related*) are like any diets: you can lose, maintain, or gain weight. Here's how you do it.

Lose Weight

Like any other eating regimen, caloric intake and portion control are important factors when it comes to weight loss. A pound of fat on your body is 3,500 stored calories—so if you think of it in terms of weight loss being a simple equation of calories in/calories out, then if you eat 500 calories less than you burn every day, after a week, you will have lost a pound of fat.

Whole, plant-based foods are your friend in this equation, as they offer the most nutrient density for the lowest amount of calories. They're also high in fiber, meaning you'll feel full instead of *hangry*.

If you're looking to shed pounds but hesitant to go on yet another diet, this kind of eating can be freeing. That's because a lot of people who ascribe to this way of life—consuming a vegan diet based around vegetables, fruit, a moderate amount of whole grains, healthy fats, and beans—don't wind up counting calories at all, which is why a whole foods diet can be like a breath of fresh air. Various doctors have different names for this way of eating, but it all boils down to approximately the same thing: eat mostly produce and legumes, and eat a lot of them. Author Joel Fuhrman, MD, for example, calls this way of eating a "nutritarian diet."

You've probably heard much of this before, so if you're eye-rolling, hang on. There's a reason this stuff is so familiar and repeated ad nauseam. Ready? *It works*. It really isn't rocket science (note that we didn't say it was *easy*, it's just not supercomplicated). The most important things to keep in mind if you want to lose weight are: eat your greens (center your meals around

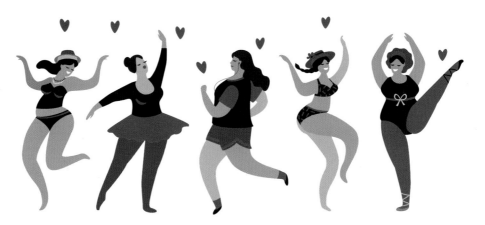

vegetables—fresh or frozen—including breakfast); keep an open mind when it comes to trying different varieties of beans, since they pack a nutritional punch; reduce oil from your diet (vegetable stock–sautéing is a thing, and it works); consume only high-quality fats, such as nuts, seeds, and avocado (but only a limited amount); make sure your bread is whole grain (don't knock Kamut until you try it!), and replace at least some of your bread with actual whole grains, such as quinoa, amaranth, or a limited amount of rice; don't drink your calories; and eat fruit for dessert (frozen bananas or mango whip up to a delish soft-serve in a high-powered blender). Leave your calorie-counting in the past and enjoy your life, goddammit. Bear in mind that all these guidelines are for weight *loss*, and are not forever, which leads us to . . . maintenance!

Maintain Weight

For weight maintenance, you should still stick to a relatively whole foods, unprocessed diet, but you no longer need to create a calorie deficit. This leaves room for a few more indulgences, so you can have that New York slice of vegan pizza a bit more often than you would if you were trying to lose weight. Again, it's all about balance. If you ever find yourself wanting to lose or gain weight, make a few simple adjustments. The base of your diet—regardless of whether you're losing, maintaining, or gaining weight—should remain pretty close to whole foods sources. To go from maintenance to weight gain, add additional calories in the form of more whole grains as well as high-quality fats (avocado, nuts, and seeds), and you'll be on your way.

Gain Weight

For a lot of men in particular, going vegan brings with it the stigma of being scrawny and skinny. If that's you, immediately flip to Chapter 8, which covers important facts about fitness and staying strong—but also know that you can healthily gain weight as a vegan, should you need or want to.

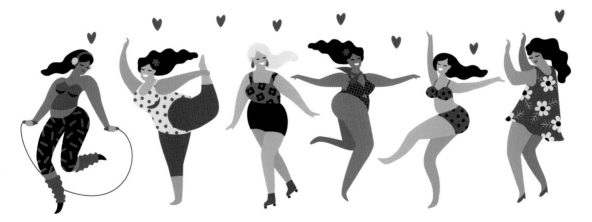

To put on muscle, you need to do two things: up your calories and your strength training. You cannot gain muscle without these two components—add more calories without exercise and you'll gain fat; exercise without a sufficient source of calories and you'll lose weight (first in the form of fat, then your body will start eating your muscles—not fun).

There are a plethora of plant-based programs, both paid and free, available online if you really want to get into the weeds of counting macros (veganfitness.com is a good place to start), but you can also go by feel. Weigh yourself once a week. Are you stagnating or losing weight? Then, up your total calories by 300 to 500 per day, focusing on increasing your healthy fats, such as nut butters, adding some plant-based protein powders (make sure there's no whey lingering in the ingredients list, as it is dairy-derived), and stepping up the amount of whole grains you consume.

Focus on strength-building exercises (such as weightlifting and calisthenics) while keeping your cardio (running, swimming, cycling, kickboxing, Zumba, etc.) to a moderate amount. It's common for those who partake in cardio-heavy exercise to tend to have the most trouble gaining weight simply because this form of exercise burns so many calories.

But Weight . . .

It's worth repeating that veganism is not a weight-loss regimen. When you go vegan, you're making the best possible choice for yourself, but also for the planet and for the animals.

You probably have figured out by now that animals' bodies are not ours to abuse or eat, so one could argue that our veganism is a way of respecting another individual's bodily integrity. No one wants to oppress another body, so why oppress our own? Body positivity—not only just accepting, but going the extra mile to in fact *love*—the vessel you are moving through this world in is, plain and simple, a political act. Choosing to feel comfortable in your skin is a vital part of self-growth, and veganism can help propel that forward. That's because, for most of us, making the decision to no longer consume animal products is a move toward authenticity and living in a continuum with our belief systems.

If you look around, you will find vegans whose bodies resemble your own; they are beautiful and sexy, as are you. This is a bold statement, but sometimes loving yourself begins by simply deciding to love yourself, and then you can focus on reframing the negative mind-set that you've spent so many years perfecting. You're eating in alignment with your values now; why not hold yourself accountable to love with an open heart, too? If you want to lose weight, or if you want to gain weight, then by all means, you can; it's your body. But along the way, do yourself a favor and be gentle. You are on a journey. You might as well enjoy it.

Mirror Image

No matter your size, you are worth celebrating. Here's how to start thinking differently about yourself when you look in the mirror, no matter what shape you are.

❑ If you find yourself whispering statements under your breath, such as "I hate myself," start to notice it. Then, every single time you do, apologize to yourself and say the opposite. This won't feel natural for a while, but do it anyway. So, say, **"I'm sorry. I don't hate you. I am learning to love you."** Do it every single time. Words are powerful, so choose them wisely. Every time you hate on yourself, you're depleting your energy and vitality.

❑ Just before you gaze at your mirror image, tell yourself that the person you are about to look at is cute. That way, instead of preparing to look at yourself with that dread or negativity already boiling over, **you can start to set yourself up for successful self-nurturing**. Do it over and over before looking at your reflection, and then once you do look, see whether you can start to find the cute, attractive, or beautiful attributes you have—perhaps gazing at yourself as someone else might, instead of letting your old demons determine your mindset.

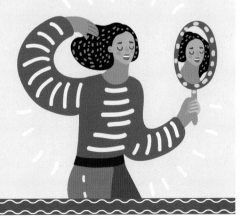

❑ **Keep a gratitude list of all the things about yourself that you appreciate**. This can include a mix of character traits and physical traits. Try to remember things most of us take for granted, including if you're ambidextrous, if you have clear skin, or if you're a good listener. If you're coming up blank, then to start, ask a trusted friend for suggestions.

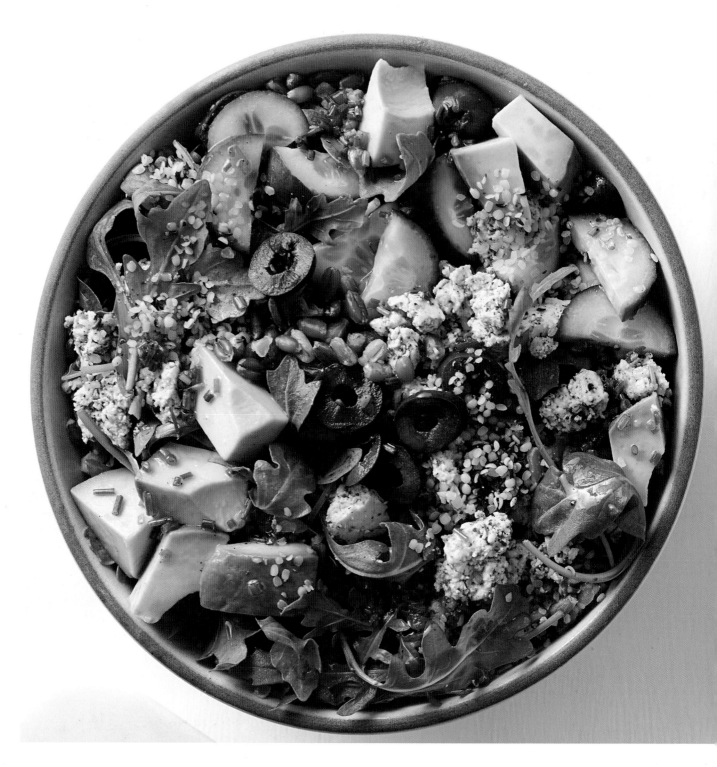

Middle Eastern Farro Salad with Avocado & Za'atar Feta

Serves 2

This filling, nutritious salad boasts hearty grains, leafy greens, a dose of vegan protein, healthy fats, and a ton of Middle Eastern–inspired flavor.

Farro:
- 1½ cups uncooked farro
- 1 teaspoon salt

Crumbled za'atar tofu feta:
- 8 ounces extra-firm tofu
- 1 tablespoon za'atar
- 1 tablespoon kalamata olive brine (reserved liquid from jarred olives)
- ½ tablespoon olive oil

Lemon-chive dressing:
- 2 tablespoons olive oil
- 2 teaspoons agave nectar
- 2 tablespoons freshly squeezed lemon juice
- ¼ teaspoon salt
- ¼ teaspoon freshly ground black pepper
- 2 tablespoons minced chives

To serve:
- 5 cups arugula
- 1 cup halved and thinly sliced cucumber
- ⅓ cup thinly sliced kalamata olives
- 1 avocado, peeled, pitted, and diced

1 **Prepare the farro:** Place farro in a medium-size pot, and cover with water. Season with salt and bring to a boil over high heat. Lower heat to a simmer and cook until farro is al dente, about 30 minutes. Drain and let cool.

2 **Prepare the crumbled za'atar tofu feta:** Press tofu between two kitchen towels to drain as much moisture as possible. In a medium bowl, crumble tofu into small pieces. Sprinkle with za'atar, then drizzle with kalamata olive brine and ½ tablespoon olive oil. Mix well to combine and refrigerate until ready to serve.

3 **Prepare the lemon-chive dressing:** In a small bowl, whisk together all dressing ingredients until thoroughly combined.

4 To assemble, in a large bowl, combine cooled farro with arugula, cucumber, kalamata olives, and 1 cup of tofu mixture. Add ⅓ cup of dressing, and gently toss. Divide among serving plates and garnish with avocado.

There's More to Life Than a Leather Couch

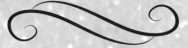

Day 15

*If you're asking, "Do I need to throw out my leather couch?" the answer is yes. Just kidding. **Kind of.***

For a new

vegan, there might be nothing more shocking than going to a friend's house and gasping at their animal-skin rug splayed across the floor. Should you step on it without a care, as everyone else seems to be doing? Or should you put together an impromptu funeral?

As with your leather belt collection, you don't need to freak out and immediately throw out all of your furniture that doesn't conform to your new way of life—your leather sofa, your wool rug, your fur throw (well, okay: maybe you can go donate that right away, since it's staggeringly cruel and remarkably easy to replace). A lot of people who start down the vegan path take a while—in many cases, years—to replace all nonvegan furnishings (and wardrobe items) with the cruelty-free counterpart. So, before you put your favorite Anthropologie loveseat on your lawn with a tear-stained sign that says "FREE!!!!" with perhaps a few too many exclamation points,

take a pause, be grateful for your ongoing journey in this crazy world, and know that in the fullness of time, all the things around you will reflect your value system. This includes your IKEA collection.

Just like anything else, veganizing your furniture and household items is actually a really fun and energizing process. The flip side of the fright and frustration of starting to recognize the universality of animal exploitation is the joy that comes with replacing old items with new ones. Once you start researching such things as eco-friendly vegan furniture, you will quickly see that there's a whole world out there, and that there is indeed a strong market for earth-friendly synthetics. As for many vegans, finding items that reflect your values and style becomes like a hobby, and for the budget-minded, there are also a ton of ethical solutions that will keep your budget as intact as your moral baseline.

When considering low-impact sofas and other furniture items that are also free of animal products, there are some overarching principles to pay attention to. What makes furniture sustainable and cruelty-free? Some things to consider are: the materials (obviously avoid leather, wool, down, and fur—but beyond that, in terms of sourcing, ask yourself whether the environmental impact is low, or maybe even nonexistent? Are the raw materials recyclable, nontoxic, and renewable?); the method of production (is it fair-trade? Is there a small carbon footprint?); as well as the finish (is it nontoxic?); life cycle (is it reusable or biodegradable?); and durability (how long will it last?).

Leather (which includes suede) is one of the most common animal products you will find on furniture. Aside from the animal torture, bear in mind that most leather production employs chromium and other very toxic chemicals in the dying and tanning processes, and it's not uncommon for that industry to also employ child labor. Instead of leather, opt for a natural fabric, such as organic cotton or linen.

Beyond just the couch itself, you'll want to make sure that your cushions are synthetic, too, and filled with a cruelty-free product instead of down—which is rife with its own set of nasty issues. Down, the softest layer of feathers closest to a duck's skin, is highly valued by manufacturers (but more highly valued by the ducks themselves) and is most often used in down jackets, comforters, and cushions (oh my!).

Most of the time, down (and other feathers) are removed when the duck or goose is being slaughtered, but birds who are part of breeding flocks, or are being raised for meat or foie gras (whereby they are force-fed through a tube that is rammed down their throat until their liver is fatty and diseased—*foie gras* literally means "fatty liver"), regularly undergo painful plucking while they are still alive. When they're plucked, the birds are lifted by their wings or legs, their legs are restrained or tied, and their feathers are ripped out of their skin (often resulting in their bodies being torn apart, leading to workers hurriedly sewing them up with needles). This is repeated about every six weeks until they are slaughtered for meat—which is, of course, way sooner than they'd die naturally (all farmed animals are killed as just babies—ranging in age from six weeks if they are birds to two to three years if they are cows). Instead of down or wool, opt for coconut fiber, bamboo, or organic cotton to fill your cushion and your conscience.

When veganizing your home, you might also consider the household products you use to clean. As we discussed in Chapter 12, animal testing is a real travesty, and these days it's easy to find household cleansers that don't rely on blinding rabbits to make sure your toilets sparkle. In addition to vegan brands you can find at a variety of stores, another animal- and environment-friendly option is to try natural cleansers, such as lemon juice (perfect for scrubbing tiles, sinks, and tubs), white vinegar (ideal for cleaning windows, chrome sink fixtures, and fridge shelves), and baking soda (mix with a little water, and you can easily scrub your counters and sink, then use any remaining powder to bake up a batch of vegan chocolate chip cookies).

Whether it's the rug beneath your feet, the cushion beneath your butt, or the cleanser beneath your sink, when it comes to choosing a cruelty-free lifestyle, home is most certainly where the heart is. If your heart is with the animals and the planet, it's easier than ever to reflect that in the place where you live and love.

Home Is Where the Heart Is

Here are some simple ideas to make your living space more eco-friendly, ethical, and cozy, all at the same time.

1 RUGS: From shag to faux sheepskin, you can find the perfect floor decor at most mainstream homewares stores or online, no animals required. Try Pottery Barn or Z Gallerie for trendy faux fur floor covers, or check out vegandesign.org or Etsy for one-of-a-kind, cruelty-free finds (if it's not clear, ask the manufacturer).

2 BEDDING: Donate the down comforter and opt for a cruelty-free covering, such as Nest Bedding's Natural Cotton Comforter. Swap your mattress for one from the vegan and eco-friendly Essentia brand, and get cozy with Boll and Branch organic cotton sheets or FlaxLinens' linen sheets.

3 FURNITURE: Home decor is mimicking the fashion industry, and vegan leather is in. Many mainstream furniture stores, such as West Elm and Wayfair, now carry vegan leather options. There are also countless linen and plant-based fabrics out there if you don't fancy the leather look. Just make sure to read the product details to ensure all materials are animal-free and synthetic.

4 PILLOWS: Rest easy at night on a cruelty-free pillow. Try Sable Sleeping's Goose Down Alternative pillows or the Non-Toxic Pillow from Avocado Green Mattress (this company makes great eco-friendly and vegan mattresses, too).

5 THROWS: For an animal-free fuzzy throw blanket, check out QBedding. Need something warmer? Cuddledown offers a machine-washable plush heated blanket made out of recycled polyester. Like vegan leather, faux fur throws are easy to find (hello, Target!), because cruelty-free is forever stylish.

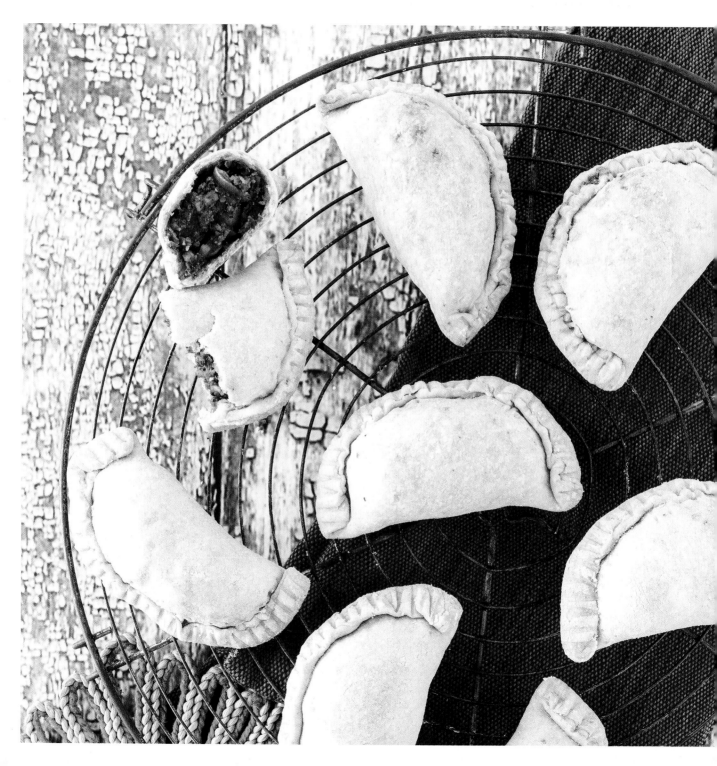

Beefy Argentinean Empanadas

Makes 12 empanadas

Whip up a platter of these mouthwatering empanadas, invite friends over, and hunker down on your leather-free couch for a night of (guilt-free) Netflix bingeing.

Dough:

1½ cups all-purpose flour, plus more for dusting
1½ cups whole wheat pastry flour
1 teaspoon salt
½ teaspoon baking powder
½ cup olive oil
¾ cup ice-cold water

Filling:

1¼ cups cooked brown lentils, or 1 (15-ounce) can, drained and rinsed
¾ cup walnuts
1 tablespoon tamari
1 teaspoon Italian seasoning
½ teaspoon smoked paprika
2 tablespoons olive oil
¾ cup finely chopped red bell pepper
1 cup finely chopped yellow onion
3 garlic cloves, minced
½ cup chopped pitted green olives
¼ cup raisins
½ teaspoon dried oregano
½ teaspoon salt
1 tablespoon tomato paste
1 tablespoon water

❶ **Prepare the dough:** In a food processor, combine flours, salt, and baking powder. Pulse until well mixed, stream in oil through the chute in the lid, and continue to pulse to incorporate. Gradually add cold water through the chute until a soft, stretchy (not sticky) dough forms.

❷ Transfer dough to a lightly floured surface and gently knead until ingredients are combined, being careful not to overwork. Divide equally into two balls and flatten each slightly into a disk. Wrap tightly with plastic wrap and refrigerate for at least 1 hour.

❸ Preheat oven to 400°F. Line a baking sheet with parchment paper.

❹ **Prepare the filling:** In a food processor, combine lentils, walnuts, tamari, Italian seasoning, and paprika. Pulse six times, or until a coarse, crumbly mixture forms. Remove from food processor and set aside.

❺ In a large sauté pan over medium-high heat, heat oil. Add bell pepper and onion and sauté until slightly softened and translucent, about 3 minutes. Add garlic, olives, raisins, oregano, salt, tomato paste, water, and lentil mixture. Lower heat to medium and cook, stirring gently, for about 3 minutes. Remove from heat.

❻ To shape empanadas, on a lightly floured surface, roll out one ball of dough to ⅛-inch thickness. Using an inverted small bowl or large biscuit cutter, cut 5-inch rounds. Add 3 tablespoons of filling to each round and fold dough in half to enclose filling. Use a fork to press and seal edges. Continue with remaining dough and filling, rerolling dough scraps to form additional rounds as needed

❼ Once all empanadas have been formed, arrange on prepared baking sheet and place in oven. Bake for 25 to 27 minutes, or until empanadas are lightly browned. Serve warm.

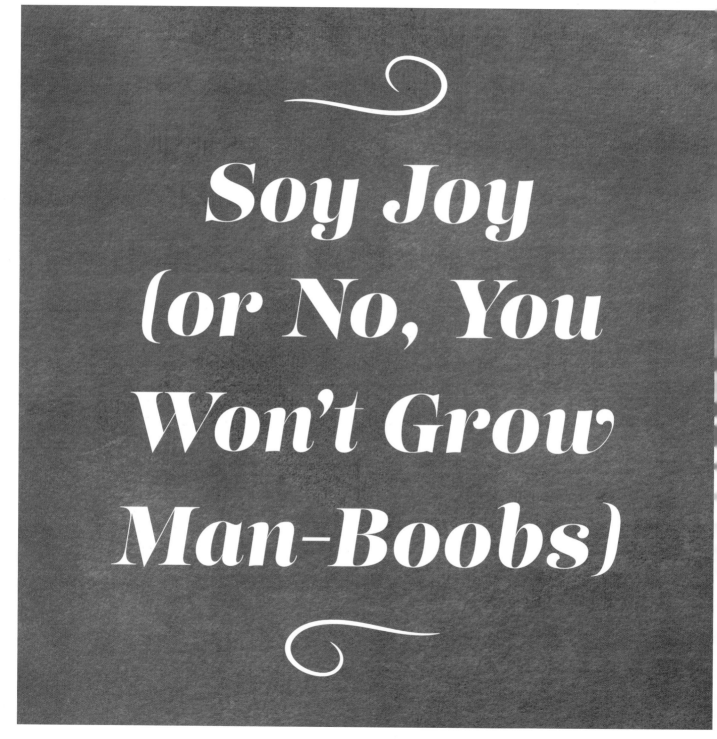

Soy Joy (or No, You Won't Grow Man-Boobs)

Day 16

*Really, **you won't.***

Soy is the

subject of some of the worst health misinformation there is (thanks, internet). But if you actually follow the science instead of the hype, you will find out that upping your intake of soy has a plethora of health benefits, including reducing the risk of (or even helping reverse) heart disease, promoting bone health, reducing hot flashes, improving cognitive function, and lowering the risk of a staggering number of cancers, including breast, prostate, lung, stomach, and colorectal.

Think about it: tofu, miso, soy milk, and tempeh have been staples of Asian cuisine for thousands of years. These nutrient-dense foods don't go away for a reason. And these traditional soy foods—as well as the more modern-day innovations of many meat analogues—are total rock stars when it comes to protein content, offering higher protein than other beans, and they are also one of the few significant plant sources of omega-3 fatty acids. Moreover, the carbohydrate in soybeans is mostly made up of oligosaccharides, sugars that help healthy bacteria grow. Soybeans also provide iron, folate, potassium, and calcium. Soy, it turns out, is extremely beneficial.

Let's get right to what the naysayers are all thinking, which is that due to the huge misperception that there's estrogen in it, soy consumption leads to man-boobs. The truth is that soy contains phytoestrogens (or plant estrogens) called isoflavones (which have both estrogenic and antiestrogenic effects), but isoflavones are not the same as estrogen—which is one of the biggest myths about soy.

So, where do man-boobs come in? Despite wide rumors, science has found no evidence cautioning men against consuming soy. On the contrary, soy can decrease the risk of prostate cancer. Most man-boobs are actually just fat on heavier men—more than 1 in 3 men are considered to be overweight, a side effect of the Standard American Diet. In short, soy products do not decrease one's perceived manliness.

It's also untrue that soy can cause breast cancer. Conversely, soy foods may, in fact, lower breast cancer risk. In Asian countries, where soy is a substantial part of the diet, breast cancer rates are significantly lower than in the United States. This fact prompted hundreds of studies, and the research suggests that soy can actually protect against the development (and recurrence of) breast cancer.

Soy's protective properties are most potent when consumed during adolescence, since that's when breast tissue is most influenced by one's diet. So, if you have (or are) a teenage girl, make sure she's (you're) getting her (your) soy, because it *actually really* does a body good—unlike dairy, which is laden with hormones and persistent inorganic pollutants that can cause a whole lot of problems for kids' hormonal balance, developing brains, and future fertility.

Like just about everything, eating closer to the source is the healthiest for us. So, eating soy in its most natural state—edamame, tofu, tempeh, and unsweetened soy milk, for example—is indeed healthier than eating an overabundance of processed soy products. That said, there is nothing unsafe about meat analogues made from isolated soy protein or soy protein concentrate (many of the studies on protein quality in soy used isolated soy proteins, in fact).

So, the next time you are confronted with someone who is still under the false illusion that soy will result in them growing man-boobs or getting breast cancer, or isn't high in protein, hold back your instinct to bang your head against the wall in intense frustration. As with so many aspects of veganism, once they look into it, they will realize that they've been living under a slab of tofu all these years and are full of misinformation as robust as the crop itself.

There is, however, one real risk you run if you choose to consume soy. When dining with friends at your favorite Japanese restaurant, you will all likely share a deliciously salty bowl of hot edamame. And all the nonvegans will eat all the edamame. In this instance, we suggest not sharing; get your own damn bowl.

Top 5 Superpowers of Soy

From its high fiber to impressive vitamin count, soy will make you feel strong and sated. Here are some of the benefits of this incredible food.

① PROTEIN

There are about 8 grams of protein in 3 ounces of organic firm tofu and up to 15 grams in some high-protein varieties. A standard 8-ounce glass of soy milk also contains 8 grams of protein (the same amount as cows' milk). Edamame contains 11 grams of protein per ½ cup, and tempeh, which is phenomenal for everything from stir-fries to vegan bacon, contains a whopping 16 grams of protein per 3-ounce serving. Eat your soy and start flexing those plant-strong muscles.

② FIBER

The daily recommended amount of fiber prescribed by the Institute of Medicine is 25 grams for women and 38 grams for men. Ninety-five percent of Americans fall short, thanks to the mass consumption of animal products, which are severely lacking in this essential nutrient. Fiber-rich soy foods, such as edamame and tempeh, contain 4 and 5 grams of fiber, respectively, per serving.

③ CHOLESTEROL-FREE

All animal products contain cholesterol, which can lead to heart disease. However, soy, like all plant-based foods, is devoid of this artery-clogging substance. Swapping in soy for high-cholesterol foods, such as cows' milk, cheese, and beef, can lower your cholesterol levels over time.

④ VITAMIN POWERHOUSE

Soy foods contain a number of essential nutrients, including B vitamins (though you still need your B_{12} supplement), potassium, and magnesium. These vitamins support a host of necessary functions in your body, from aiding muscle contractions to fighting fatigue to keeping bones strong. Supplement your daily multivitamin and pop a few edamame, or savor a delicate miso soup to power your body with these incredible micronutrients.

⑤ CANCER-KILLER

Okay, not exactly. But it can reduce the risk of hormone-dependent cancers. Soy contains phytoestrogens, which are plant-based estrogens that bind to estrogen receptors and can actually block this hormone from wreaking havoc on the body. Regular soy consumption has been linked to a decrease in risk of prostate, colon, and breast cancer in numerous studies.

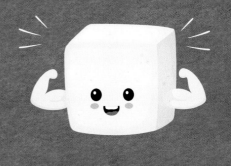

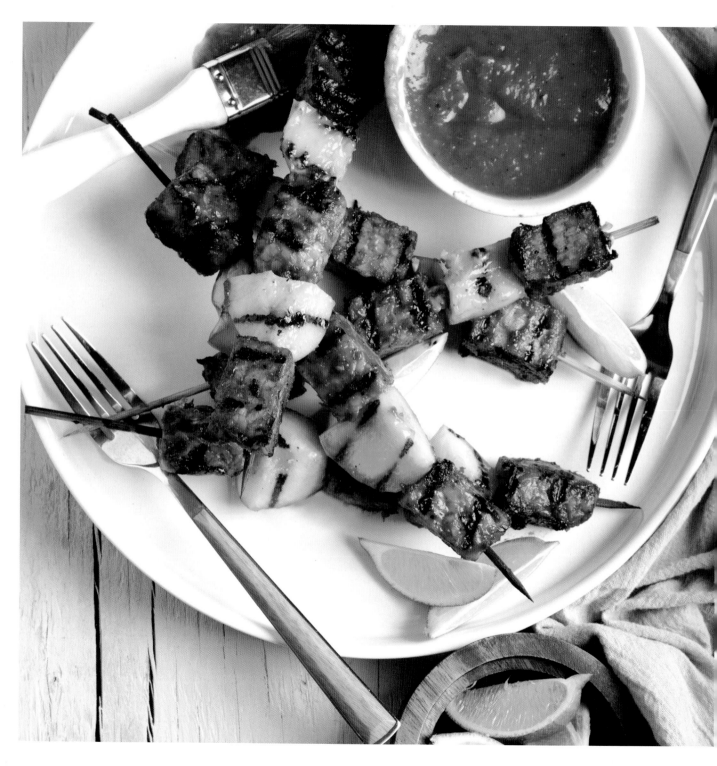

Grilled Peach & Tempeh Kebabs

Makes 6 skewers

What do you call tender, meaty morsels of tempeh plus chunks of juicy peaches all glazed in a sticky-sweet peach-infused barbecue sauce? Soy good!

Glaze:

1 tablespoon coconut oil
2 garlic cloves, chopped
½ medium-size white onion, roughly chopped
1 peach, peeled, pitted, and diced
2 tablespoons tomato paste
2 tablespoons cider vinegar
3 tablespoons pure maple syrup
1 tablespoon vegan Worcestershire sauce
½ teaspoon salt
¼ teaspoon ground allspice
¼ teaspoon freshly ground black pepper
⅛ teaspoon cayenne pepper
3 tablespoons water

Kebabs:

1 (8-ounce) package tempeh, cubed into 18 pieces
1 tablespoon coconut oil
1 peach, pitted and diced
Oil for barbecue or grill pan

1 Prepare the glaze: In a large saucepan, heat oil. Add garlic and onion and cook for 5 minutes, or until soft. Add peach and cook for another 3 minutes to soften. Add remaining glaze ingredients and cook for 5 to 8 minutes over medium heat, stirring occasionally. Transfer to blender or food processor and purée until smooth.

2 Prepare the kebabs: Soak wooden skewers in warm water for 10 minutes. Place tempeh in a bowl, coat with peach glaze, and marinate for 30 minutes. Preheat barbecue or large grill pan and brush with oil.

3 Alternate three cubes of tempeh and two of diced peach on each skewer. Grill, brushing often with peach glaze, for 4 to 5 minutes per side, or until grill marks form. Serve warm.

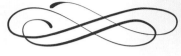

Friends & Parents & Sweeties, Oh My!

Day 17

*It would be nice if your beloved ones went vegan, too, but that's their choice. And there are ways you can support them **while remaining true to yourself**.*

There's this

funny thing about going vegan in that once people make the switch, they often go through a period of time where they start to see—as if suddenly with a bright, shining spotlight—how carelessly society has acclimated to the billions of ways animals are exploited. This can be a jarring moment, and though we can't promise you won't have one bad day where you'll find yourself standing in front of a corner hotdog stand crying, "WHYYYYYY?!?!," those rough patches do pass—leading the way to a deeper, more meaningful, and more joyous life based on a foundation of self-actualization, palate-pleasing new cuisines, and thoughtful discernment (cognitive dissonance is seriously overrated).

Somewhere around this time, a second layer of "WTF?" kicks in: the realization that on some level,

we no longer share the same common ground as our meat-eating friends/partners/spouses/parents/kids/coworkers/baristas.

Does this mean you need to break up with the people in your life who aren't vegan? Nope, it doesn't (unless you want to—in which case, *you do you*), but it might be useful to have a few extra tools in your kit so that you can best navigate the social aspects of this whole new world, especially as it impacts your close relationships.

First things first: not everyone is going to go vegan when you do. The good people whom you care about and who care about you might never go vegan, and that doesn't mean you can't continue to have a deep, meaningful relationship with them. Just as you are on your own journey, others are their own journey, too. And though learning the ropes when it comes to healthful communication tactics is sometimes a complex and multifaceted process, we can all but guarantee that nobody is going to go vegan by your battering them over the head with a seitan drumstick (better to just eat the drumstick and watch them drool over it).

That doesn't mean, however, that you should ever hide, minimize, or apologize for your veganism. In fact, we recommend you wear it proudly—even if it sometimes makes others uncomfortable. That discomfort is theirs, not yours. People frequently react strongly—and defensively—when there is a vegan in their midst, especially if that person is a new vegan who they knew before the transition occurred. Being on the other side of this will become easier for you to bear witness to, but try to not let it get you down. Being a kind, thoughtful, rational vegan who can hold space for your friends' questions or processes is key, and if they are combative or passive-aggressive with you, all you need to say is "This kind of eating really works for me." End of story.

Any discomfort your friends might be feeling (and maybe even taking out on you) is really a reflection of their own personal rising anxieties. There is no reason to eat animals; even the most defensive meat-eater likely knows that deep down, but we are deeply conditioned to act otherwise, and there are a lot of moving parts at play. This is a struggle for a lot of people, and since we're not always the most tactful or kind species, sometimes the result is plain, old-fashioned meanness. Obviously, you should never spend time with anyone who is being a jerk to you, so if that happens, use your cute new vegan boots to saunter on out of the room; just know that if

someone is putting you down because you're vegan, it's on them and their conscience.

That said, for a lot of new vegans, the question of whether their partners or family should go vegan lingers. And there is no one right answer. Many vegans who are partnered with another vegan are adamant that they could never be with a meat-eater (that's called being a *vegansexual*), but for newbies whose partners have not yet joined them on the plant side, it can be more complex.

Different people work this out differently, and whatever you decide is your bottom line is exactly spot on and doesn't need to be second-guessed; you should set and keep boundaries that you're comfortable with. Assuming you are in a healthy relationship where communication feels safe, discussing your veganism—and your evolving comfort zones when it comes to things like sharing a fridge that also stores animal products—can and should be a productive and mutually supportive dialogue.

You will learn, over time, what works and what doesn't. Give yourself (and your partner/roommates/parents) permission to change, and don't put anyone else on a timeline. As hard as it is, have compassion for them. In your prevegan days, you, too, would have felt a little stymied if someone very close to you changed their lifestyle, leaving you back in the old one all by yourself.

Having discussions about and advocating for veganism is a very individual process; there is no one right way to fight for the cause, or to show people how amazing it is to ditch animal products.

Given the multitude of reasons to go vegan (optimal health, well-being, performance, environmental sustainability, animal rights, and social justice, to name a few), you have a ton of options when it comes to conversation-starters specifically tailored to the unique person you're speaking with.

So, if you're talking with a football fan, you might point out that fifteen members of the Tennessee Titans went plant-based to improve their game. If you're speaking with a college student majoring in philosophy, you might question why the hell they chose philosophy as a major. Just kidding—you might actually ask whether they've ever read *Animal Liberation* by Peter Singer, a famed ethicist who is often referred to as the grandfather of the animal-rights movement, and one of *Time*'s Most Influential People of the last century. If you're hanging out with someone who is switching to an electric car because of their care for the planet, you might ask for a ride, then work into the conversation how animal agriculture is responsible for 18 percent of greenhouse gas emissions, which is more than the combined exhaust from all transportation. Just try your best not to sound righteous, which is frequently only possible when these types of conversations are said using "I" statements ("For sure, I'm trying to do what I can for the environment. It's blowing my mind how much food choices can affect climate change"). Focusing on yourself and your own transformation will have a better effect than pedantically talking *at* someone and lecturing them. Better yet, offer them a vegan cookie. Or hand over that seitan drumstick.

Finally, it's worth acknowledging that sometimes—in fact, frequently—the people closest to you won't go vegan, and learning to accept that and not put all your egg replacer in one fair-trade, handwoven basket is superimportant. Being vegan is one thing, but if you want to be an advocate for the cause, look beyond just the places where you live and love. There's a whole world out there full of people who are ready and eager to talk with you about veganism. It just might not be your parents.

Finally, veganism will quickly become your favorite part of you, and will absolutely, undoubtedly lead you to a new slew of awesome people who are as passionate as you are about Instagram-worthy vegan cupcakes, coffee shops that don't charge extra for nondairy milk, and animal liberation. Just be you in all of your vegan glory, and be open to the wonder and importance of vegan community. You have a whole world waiting for you. This is the time to grow.

Shared Spaces

For vegans who cohabitate with meat-eaters, it might be helpful
for everyone involved to have some simple ground rules in place.
Here are a few possible ways of negotiating your shared spaces.

❏ Keep your kitchen vegan, but **don't micromanage your partner's/roommates'/ parents' choices** when you're dining out or at friends' houses.

❏ **Keep one specific shelf in the fridge**—or one set of pots and pans—exclusively for nonvegan (or vegan) food.

❏ Choose one day a week, or several days per week, to **go vegan as a family** or a unit—such as weekdays only—and then, on the other days, do your own thing.

❏ Create a ground rule that **veganism will not be discussed over shared meals**, because in that setting, it can create tenseness or defensiveness.

❏ Agree that **all household cleansers will be cruelty-free**, and offer to be in charge of picking those up each time.

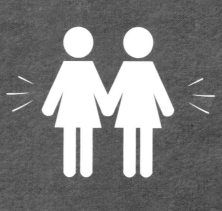

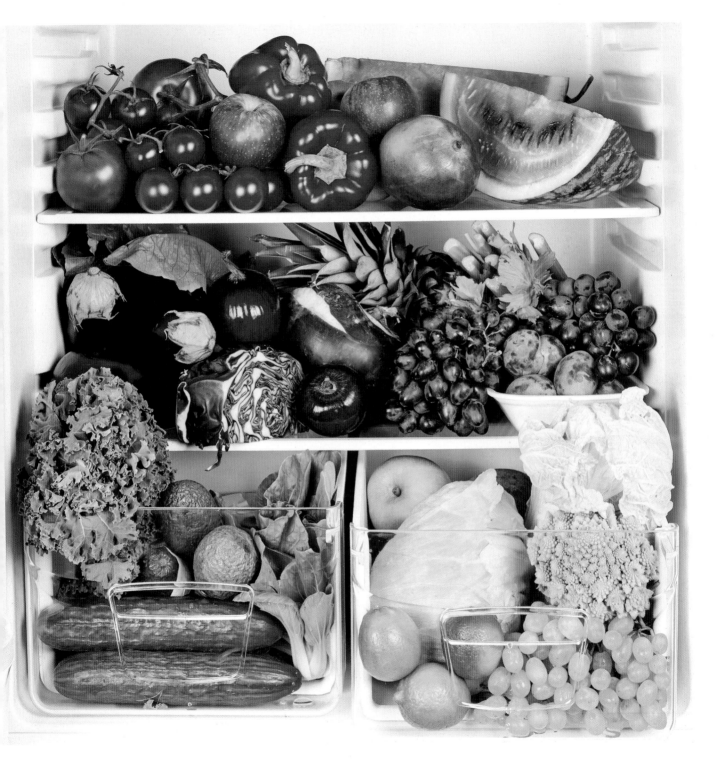

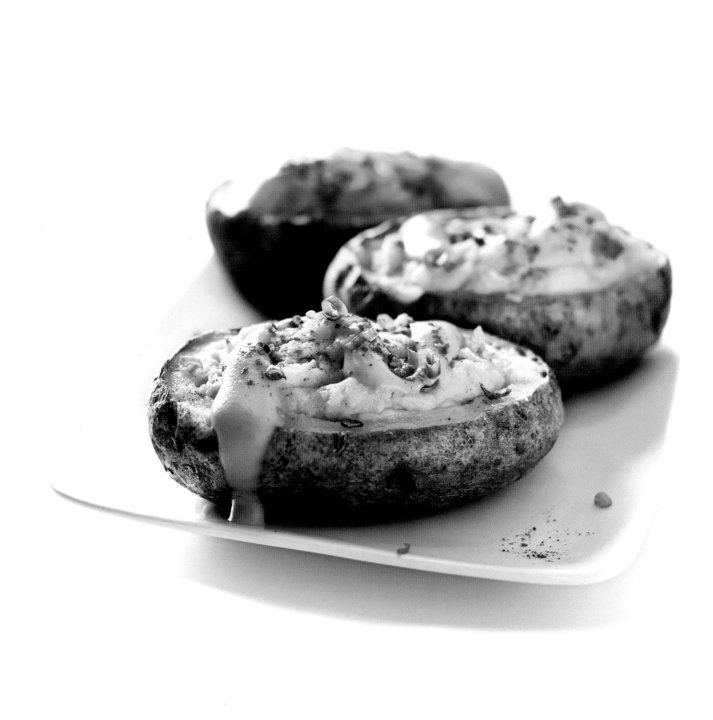

Cheesy Twice-Baked Potatoes

Satisfy everyone at the dinner table with these crowd-pleasing entrée potatoes. Pro tip: add steamed broccoli to the filling to sneak in some healthy veggies for the kids (okay, and the adults).

Baked potatoes:

8   large russet potatoes, scrubbed
2   tablespoons olive oil
¼   teaspoon salt

Cheddar cheese sauce:

⅓   cup vegan butter
¼   cup chopped onion
1   cup chopped, peeled potato
¼   cup chopped carrot
½   teaspoon minced garlic
1   teaspoon smoked paprika
1   teaspoon salt

1   cup water
¼   cup raw cashews
⅛   teaspoon Dijon mustard
1   tablespoon freshly squeezed lemon juice

Mashed potato filling:

¼   cup vegan butter
¼   cup unsweetened vegan milk
1   teaspoon salt
1   teaspoon freshly ground black pepper, plus more for garnish
1   cup vegan sour cream
6   scallions, thinly sliced

1 **Prepare the potatoes:** Preheat oven to 375°F. Place potatoes on a baking sheet and rub with 1 tablespoon of oil and salt. Pierce each potato several times with a fork. Bake for 70 minutes, or until soft.

2 **Prepare the Cheddar cheese sauce:** In a sauté pan over medium heat, melt butter. Add onion and cook for 5 minutes. Add chopped potato, carrot, garlic, paprika, and salt and sauté for 5 minutes. Add water and bring to a boil. Cover pan and simmer for 20 minutes, or until vegetables are very soft. In a high-powered blender, combine cashews, mustard, lemon juice, and chopped potato mixture. Process until cheese sauce is smooth, then set aside.

3 Remove baked potatoes from oven and cut in half lengthwise. Using a spoon, carefully scoop out flesh from skins into a medium bowl, leaving a ¼-inch layer of potato. Brush potato shells with remaining olive oil and return to oven to bake for 15 minutes.

4 **Prepare the mashed potato filling:** Mash reserved potato flesh with butter, milk, salt, and pepper. Fold in half of sour cream, half of cheese sauce, and half of scallions. Fill each baked potato skin with mashed potato mixture. Top with a dollop of cheese sauce and drizzle with sour cream.

5 Bake loaded potato skins for 15 minutes, until thoroughly heated and tops are browned. Garnish with remaining scallions, sour cream, and pepper and serve warm.

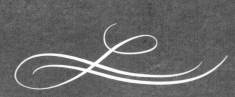

This Whole
Damn Climate
Change Thing

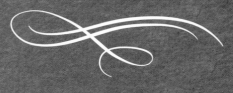

Day 18

You may recycle and use your own canvas bags (hurrah!), but still, climate change is more dire than you think—and **the single best way to fight it is to go vegan.**

We have all

known someone who is outspoken about the environment—instrumental in ensuring community compost bins are available to all, constantly picking up bottles and cans from sidewalks, or heavily involved in their college-wide protests to divest the campus's endowment of fossil fuel stocks—yet is a self-proclaimed "meathead" who starts off the day with sausage and ends it with steak. Then there are the straw-protestors who are absolutely irate that the nearby restaurant hasn't yet banned these sea turtle–torturing plastic tubes, ignoring the fact that the restaurant itself serves sea animals.

Of course, all of that is indeed a bit self-righteous. Suffice it to say, even know-it-alls like us who have learned all the ways meat production is destroying the planet are on our own journeys of self-betterment and social justice, and should always remain open to stepping up our own game. For those of us who care

about the health of this planet we all share, humility is an important value, since everyone—including not-yet-vegan environmentalists—need to show up for this quickly deteriorating planet we share. So, we need to work together. We are the world. We are the children. (You're welcome for the earworm.)

Truly, the impact that animal production is having on our planet could not possibly be more severe. Agriculture is responsible for about a quarter of all global anthropogenic greenhouse gas emissions; animal agriculture accounts for 80 percent of this. Think about it: in the United States, more than ten billion land animals are slaughtered for food annually—with your average American consuming 200 pounds of meat each year. This amount of meat production carries with it a significant amount of resources. Here is a glimpse into how:

❑ **One pound of beef requires 1,800 gallons of water**—the equivalent of 105 eight-minute showers a day.

- **Animal agriculture is the leading cause of deforestation**—in 2018, 30 million acres of tropical rainforest were lost (a rate of 43 football fields a minute).
- **Livestock take up to 83 percent of farmland** but provide only 18 percent of calories worldwide.
- **Two billion tons of manure a year from US livestock alone (or 12 billion pounds each day) are produced**—a significant portion of which is stored in open lagoons of literal shit. Then, along with the antibiotic residues, chemicals, and bedding, the manure is sprayed on farmlands as fertilizer, delivering the *E. coli* that prompts recalls of your romaine lettuce.
- **Over a 100-year period, the greenhouse gas methane has over 25 times the impact on the earth as carbon dioxide**—and the biggest contributor of methane in the United States is livestock and the waste they produce.

It's pretty evident from these startling numbers that animal agriculture puts an enormous strain on the planet's land, energy, and water resources. Look at it this way: 16 percent of the world's freshwater, one-third of the ice-free land surface, and a third of worldwide grain production are used for the whopping fifty-six billion land animals raised for food. Replacing beef with plants would bring the yearly CO2e amount down by 96 percent—from 1,984 pounds per average American to just 73 pounds of CO2e.

Daunting, huh? But that also means that each of us holds within our power the ability to vote with our dollars and become much more conscious about the impacts of our consumption choices.

A vegan, as you know by now, is someone who eats the plants that grow, and . . . that's about it. A nonvegan ate the plants that grew that were then fed to the animals who needed to convert the plants into muscle, then were slaughtered, and then their bodies were transported and packaged. Phew, that's a lot of resources right there!

Plus, the meat-eater who ate that animal who used those resources is only consuming a part of the animal's body, thereby only getting a small part of the energy input that they could have obtained had they eaten the plants directly. When you consider the land, water, and effort needed to grow the plants that become animal feed, the middleman—the animal we eat—is entirely unnecessary. Beyond unnecessary, by continuing to partake in a system reliant on animal production, we become complicit in an oppressive system that is responsible for the greatest threat to humankind in history. So, yeah, let's not do that. There are other ways.

By the way, back-pocket this for when some smart-ass says to you that "plants have feelings, too." Just respond by saying that if they honestly believe that—despite the fact that plants lack a central nervous system—then they definitely shouldn't consume animals, because of the huge amount of plants that animals eat before getting slaughtered themselves. Then, roll your eyes. Then, eat a vegan cookie, knowing that that cookie is basically saving the world.

Sustainable Swaps

The numbers behind how much waste is created by everyday, single-use items are staggering. Be a part of the solution by switching throwaway goods with reusable versions.

EACH YEAR, WE WASTE:	INSTEAD, TRY THIS:
185 billion plastic straws	Stainless-steel straws (try Greens Steel)
35 billion plastic water bottles	Bamboo or stainless-steel water bottles (try Klean Kanteen)
40 billion plastic utensils	Bamboo utensil sets (try To-Go Ware)
50 billion paper coffee cups	Reusable glass tumblers (try Joco Cups)
269,000 tons of plastic takeout containers	Stainless-steel bento boxes (try ECOlunchbox)

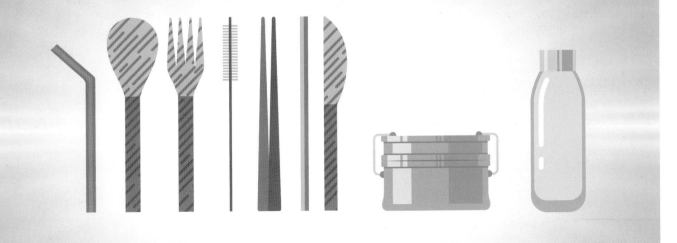

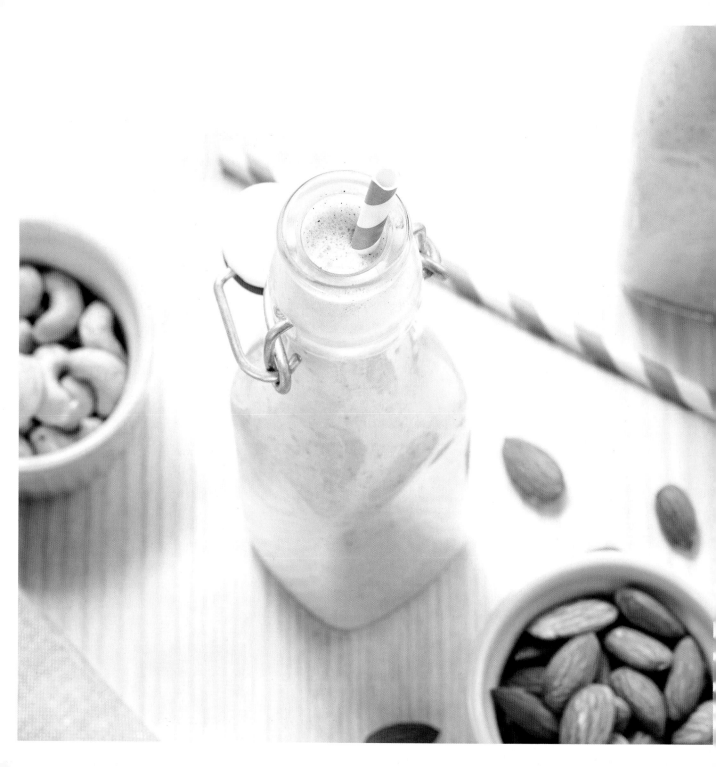

Easy Homemade Vegan Milks

Making your own plant-based milk is supersimple and environmentally friendly—not only are you avoiding all the emissions associated with the dairy industry, but you're cutting out wasteful packaging to boot! Plus, you get to experiment with different flavor combinations. Win-win-win!

Chocolate Walnut Milk

1   cup walnuts
1   tablespoon raw cacao powder
3   pitted dates
4   cups water

In a high-speed blender, combine all ingredients and blend until smooth. Strain through a nut-milk bag or cheesecloth, transfer to a pitcher, and refrigerate.

Golden Sesame Milk

1   cup white sesame seeds
½   teaspoon ground turmeric
½   teaspoon ground ginger
3   tablespoons coconut sugar
4   cups water

In a high-speed blender, combine all ingredients and blend until smooth. Strain through a nut-milk bag or cheesecloth, transfer to a pitcher, and refrigerate.

Horchata Oat Milk

1   cup rolled oats
1   teaspoon ground cinnamon
1   teaspoon pure vanilla extract
1½ tablespoons agave nectar
4   cups water

In a high-speed blender, combine all ingredients and blend until smooth. Strain through a nut-milk bag or cheesecloth, transfer to a pitcher, and refrigerate.

Strawberry Cashew Milk

1   cup raw cashews
2   cups fresh strawberries
1½   tablespoons pure maple syrup
4   cups water

In a high-speed blender, combine all ingredients and blend until smooth. Strain through a nut-milk bag or cheesecloth, transfer to a pitcher, and refrigerate.

~~~~~~

Vanilla Bean Almond Milk

1   cup raw almonds
1   vanilla bean, scraped
⅛   teaspoon sea salt
2   tablespoons sugar
4   cups water

In a high-speed blender, combine all ingredients and blend until smooth. Strain through a nut-milk bag or cheesecloth, transfer to a pitcher, and refrigerate.

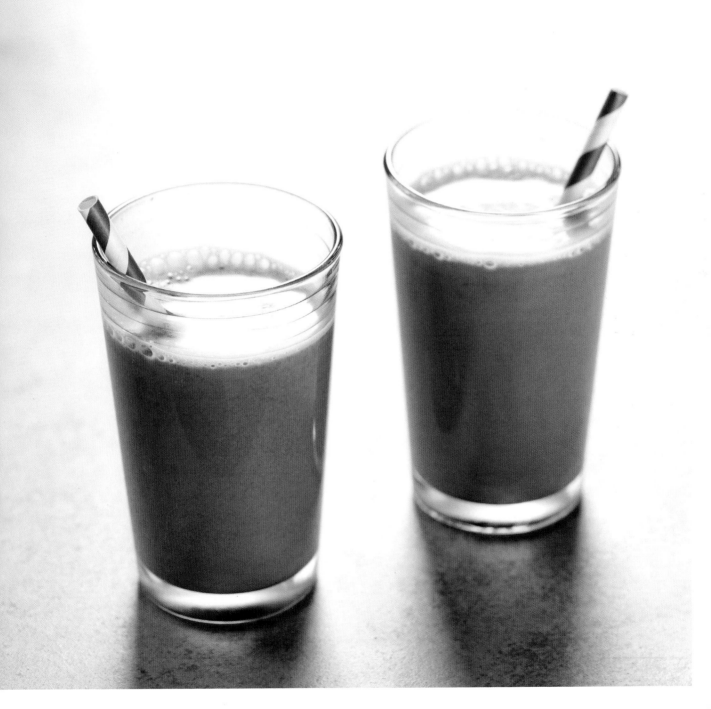

The Elephant in the Room: Failure

Day 19

*The weight of new things can indeed be scary, so **let's just focus on today.***

At first, the

word *vegan* can feel prohibitively permanent. It is a vulnerable thing to join the plant side when it can feel as though you're leaving others in your life behind. Plus, in this day and age of social media—with everything from our breakfast choices to our Saturday night movie plans being so public—being witnessed as a new vegan can feel like there's accountability that you're not ready to take on.

The unfortunate truth is that just as many of us know a few vegans, we might also know at least one ex-vegan. And even though the old joke has truth to it—"How do you know if someone is vegan? They won't stop telling you!"—there are few people louder than *ex*-vegans. It seems that, for the most part, those who have tried and for whatever reason, stopped or failed, *really want you to know about it*.

Like anything else, there are reasons why veganism doesn't stick for everyone—and the good news is that they are *prettttttty* easy to unpack:

- ❑ **Equating food restriction with veganism.** Food restriction—such as the 500-calorie-a-day diet, various types of fasting, or cutting out big categories of food—is usually unsustainable, period.
- ❑ **A lack of high-quality fat.** Adding high-quality fat—such as nuts, seeds, and avocados—to your meals helps to keep you sated for longer, and helps your body absorb important nutrients.
- ❑ **Food addiction: it's a thing.** Generally speaking, most people need 66 days for their body to adjust to a new habit, meaning people might experience cravings for animal foods for that period of time. Stay strong and trust

your body. It will adjust and you won't think twice about bacon (unless it's PigOut vegan bacon chips).

- **A nonsupportive environment.** If a new vegan has to struggle with lack of community (plus difficulty with sharing living spaces with non-vegans), they could conceivably throw in the towel. Finding and fostering safe spaces is vital to long-term veganism—and it doesn't have to mean those people will necessarily be in your family or immediate circle of friends (though it's certainly nice when they are).
- **Unexpected or unwanted weight loss or weight gain.** Although we cover this in Chapter 14, a reason people might stop being vegan is that they are still acclimating themselves to new food. It's easy to be and stay vegan, but there are sometimes a few adjustments one needs to make, such as adding or removing fat, or adding or removing grains.

Another reason someone might stop being vegan is that they are simply overwhelmed. Ever wanted to see a movie, but didn't know how to choose which one, so instead you stay in and scroll through Instagram all night while drinking a half-can of flat soda or beer that was in the fridge since last week? Sometimes, too many options can, ironically, leave us stuck in indecision, and for veganism, that might mean jumping ship. Here's some advice: take your veganism one day at a time. You can also interpret that as one latte, one meal, or one shoe-shopping trip at a time. For any big life move you make—however obvious, fun, and soul-satisfying—there is usually at least one "holy shit!" day, where it all feels too much. Listen closely: part of that feeling is coming face-to-face for the first time with the reality of your choices for the past however-many years. For a lot of vegans, that's really the source of the overwhelm. It can be daunting, to say the least, to become consciously aware of all of the abuse and damage we were partaking in during our years of ignorantly consuming animal products because society—and our well-intentioned parents—told us to.

But veganism is about abundance, not deprivation. It's about opportunity, not scarcity. Like any other choice, veganism requires a positive mind-set—especially in the instances where you are the only one in your circle who is vegan. When dining out, for example, most of the time the restaurants are going to have ample vegan options; at the very least, the chef will be able to make something for you with a simple substitution. But in the case where you are at one of the fewer and fewer places where the server thinks *vegan* is pronounced "vay-gun" and means you are a fan of Suzanne Vega, then just take a deep breath. Know that even though this is an incredibly frustrating moment, it will pass, and all of this will later be chalked up to information. If the restaurant is actually not vegan-friendly at all, then do the best you can while you're there; that means different things to different people, and there is no one right answer. If all else fails, order the salad and fries (they're probably vegan), focus on the company you're with (not what they're eating), enjoy the conversation (as best you can), and look forward to a late-night drive-thru gallivant for the Impossible Whopper (hold the cheese) later on.

Avoid situations like this in the future by checking out the menu online or, if need be, contacting the restaurant ahead of time to make sure there's something for you to eat; working with your family to choose a place that has more options; and using the handy-dandy tool of Yelp reviews and the like to make the case later to please *up* their vegan game. Remember that in the grand scheme of things, these frustrating moments will be way fewer and far between in comparison to the amount of times you will be pleasantly surprised by the vegan options.

There are also going to be people who are intrigued by veganism but nervous that their overbearing mother will be deeply offended on Easter if they don't eat the iconic family ham. Don't throw the baby (animal) out with the bathwater; if there are a few instances in your life surrounding food that you can't imagine how you'll handle as a vegan, then just trust that by the time Easter (or whatever) rolls around, you'll know what to do—and what you'll do is *the best you can*. At the end of the day,

the only person you have to answer to is yourself. At the same time, since veganism is ultimately about compassion, remember to be compassionate to yourself, too. That's not an excuse to go "hog wild" and regularly compromise your ethics—nor is it an excuse to be lazy or complacent when it comes to your food choices—but if you are honestly doing the best you can in a situation, and you feel proud of your decisions, then you are doing just fine.

Labels are both superimportant and not at all important. The point is to learn about the truth of what's happening behind closed doors to animals, how our food choices are affecting the planet, and all the ways animal consumption is making us sicker and sicker—and then to act accordingly. There are billions of lives on the line—yours included—so, even if you're on the fence about what you can do about it, doing nothing is really not an option. The great news is that a remarkable synergy is created by getting animal exploitation out of your life; it turns out that it's the best thing you can do for yourself, for the people of the world, for the earth we all share, and for the animals. However you want to label or not label yourself, or post about publicly or keep on the down low, is entirely up to you.

Leaning In

To combine a couple of clichés, don't let the exceptions swallow the rule, but at the same time, don't let the perfect be the enemy of the good. Here are some possible options for how to start on that road to 100 percent plant-based.

- ❑ **Consider "reducetarianism."** Coined by activist Brian Kateman, reducetarianism is the practice of eating fewer animal products. This is perfect for your combative uncle who just got diagnosed with heart disease and knows he needs to stop eating so much meat but is not interested in the "all-or-nothing" approach.

- ❑ **Join the "Meatless Mondays" movement.** Cut out meat (at least) one day a week. The goal of this initiative, founded in 2003, is to reduce meat consumption by 15 percent. The Meatless Monday movement has been wildly successful, with school districts, restaurants, and even some cities resolving to follow it.

- ❑ **Be "Vegan Until 6."** Created by famed food writer Mark Bittman, this is basically exactly what you think it is: go vegan until 6 p.m. If, for whatever reason, you feel you're unable to make a full commitment, just do the best you can after 6 p.m.

- ❑ **Call yourself a "flexitarian."** This is a viable choice for people who aren't quite ready to try the word *vegan* on for size, but are otherwise totally on board with veganism. It basically means that you're more or less vegan, but you occasionally, for whatever reason, stray.

- ❑ **Be "veganish" instead of vegan.** Bestselling author Kathy Freston's *The Book of Veganish* came out in 2016, and was specifically geared toward "socially aware teens and young adults" who are more or less ready to take the vegan leap, but understand that we live in an imperfect world, so they leave room for imperfect choices (which, by the way, full-throttle veganism does, too, since veganism is not about perfection—but some people feel more comfortable with a less finite-sounding word attached to their behavior, allowing them to let go of any qualms about ordering the honey-laden latte at their local coffee shop).

Baja Cauliflower Tacos with Mango Relish

Makes 12 tacos

This play on the classic Southern California fish taco is crispy, familiar, and sure to become an instant new favorite.

Mango relish:
2½ cups finely diced mango
1 jalapeño pepper, seeded and minced
2 tablespoons chopped fresh cilantro
1½ tablespoons freshly squeezed lime juice
¼ teaspoon salt

Tacos:
2 cups chickpea flour
½ cup coarse cornmeal
2 teaspoons baking powder
1 teaspoon dulse flakes
1 teaspoon ground cumin
1 teaspoon chili powder
1 teaspoon garlic powder
½ teaspoon salt
½ teaspoon freshly ground black pepper
2¼ cups (about 1½ bottles) Mexican lager-style beer

1 head cauliflower, cut into bite-size florets
4 cups vegetable oil, for frying
½ teaspoon salt
12 corn tortillas, grilled or toasted
2½ cups shredded red cabbage
1 cup Chipotle Mayonesa (recipe follows)

1 Prepare the mango relish: In a large bowl, combine all relish ingredients and refrigerate for 1 hour to allow flavors to meld. Relish will keep in refrigerator for 3 to 4 days.

2 Prepare the tacos: In a large bowl, whisk together chickpea flour, cornmeal, baking powder, dulse flakes, cumin, chili powder, garlic powder, salt, and pepper. Add beer and whisk well. The batter should resemble a slightly thick pancake batter. If too thick, add more beer, 1 tablespoon at a time, until desired consistency is reached. Toss cauliflower into batter to coat evenly.

3 In a large pot over medium heat, bring oil to 350°F. Working in batches of three, carefully drop battered cauliflower into oil, one at a time, and fry for 3 to 4 minutes, or until golden brown. Using tongs, remove cauliflower and place on a paper towel–lined plate to absorb excess oil, then sprinkle with salt. Repeat with remaining cauliflower.

4 To assemble tacos, place three to five cauliflower florets in the center of each tortilla. Top each with shredded cabbage, Chipotle Mayonesa, and mango relish.

Chipotle Mayonesa

Makes 2 cups

2   cups store-bought vegan mayonnaise
½   teaspoon dry mustard
1   teaspoon salt
2   teaspoons freshly squeezed lime juice
1   teaspoon cider vinegar
2   teaspoons agave nectar
2   whole canned chipotle peppers in adobo sauce, plus 1 teaspoon adobo sauce, pureed

In a bowl, whisk together all ingredients. Transfer to a mason jar and refrigerate until ready to use.

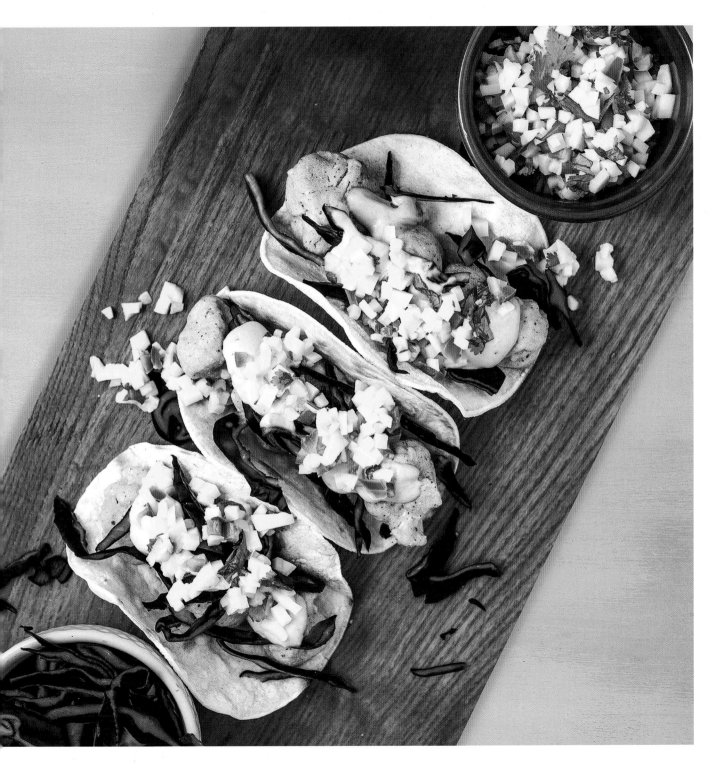

Factory Farming: It Really Is as Bad as They Say?

Day 20

*Yes. **Factory farming is an example of humanity at its worst**. It's cruel, unnecessary, and unsustainable. It's also on its way out.*

Factory farming—which is the source of virtually all meat—was created to provide an "efficient" way of keeping supply up with the demand for meat as the population boomed. Since then, it has not only met demand, but increased it. It's not efficient and it's definitely not pretty, but we'll try to make this go fast. Because to present a full-picture view of veganism, we simply have to talk about animal agriculture. Pull up a chair and pop a Xanax; we're in this together.

It's astonishing to think about the billions and billions of animals who are bred and slaughtered for our food system. Worldwide, a mind-bending seventy billion per year are reared. That number is for land animals alone, and doesn't even count the trillions of fish and other sea animals who are killed each year. In the United States, nine billion land animals are slaughtered annually for our food. That number is still impossible for us to wrap our heads around, so let's break it down further.

Every day, that's 24,657,534 land animals.

Every single second around the clock, that's 285 living beings.

If you read with an average speed, that means that since you started reading this chapter, about 19,950 land animals were killed.

All of these animals are, of course, individuals with a will to live. They are thinking, feeling beings with social circles and emotions, and they exhibit great fear as they go into the kill line.

For those of us who have been lucky enough to connect with an individual farmed animal, such as a goat, cow, pig, chicken, or turkey—perhaps during a visit to a sanctuary, where rescued animals live out the rest of their lives with dignity—these numbers are especially heartbreaking. At a sanctuary, cows who were initially raised for beef frolic and form rich social lives. Pigs run as fast as they can when it's time to eat (many love an apple snack), then they cool off in the mud because they lack functional sweat glands and doing so helps them regulate their body temperature (by the way, it's been proven that pigs are smarter than three-year-old humans). Roosters boldly protect their flock of hens. Stories like these are unending, and animal behaviorists are aware of the deep, complex thoughts of these beings whom we so easily dismiss as "there for our use." But what happens when we strip away the unjustified excuses and see these beings as individuals who feel? What we are left with, quite frankly, is a human-made atrocity (the hope in that statement is that if we made it, we have the power to change it, too).

Factory farming initially boomed after World War II as a way to continue to feed animal products to the growing masses. Factories were created to meet the demand for commercially produced meats because it was the only way to greatly reduce the amount of land that animals had access to (not to mention the fact that animals who roam consume more food and water—thus also requiring more labor and expense—than animals who are confined to small spaces).

That's when everything changed, and the interlocking issues of oppression, in fact, run deep; animal agriculture is like an elaborate, connected web of exploitation. You can't have veal without dairy, for example (if a dairy cow—who is systemically repeatedly inseminated and impregnated—gives birth to a male calf, he is of no use to the dairy industry directly). And since he wasn't created to be a beef cow, he is traditionally made to be anemic so that his flesh is considered supple, thus the "delicacy," veal. Similarly, since all parts of the animals are used, the skin of animals raised for food becomes leather, the bones are often used for such products as gelatin, duck and goose feathers might become down, and chicken feathers could be fed back to chickens as cheap feed. This is arguably a very efficient system indeed, but it's also grossly unsustainable—since animal agriculture is responsible for more greenhouse gas emissions than the exhaust of the entire travel sector combined—as well as appallingly unethical.

The routine abuse and torture of animals on factory farms is hard to wrap one's head around, but it's happening around the clock, and has somehow become so entrenched in our society today that we don't even think about it. If we did, here are a few of the things we'd learn.

Chickens Used for Eggs

Some activists say that chickens used for egg production arguably have it the worst, since the egg industry is egregiously cruel and every aspect of their short lives hideous at best. First of all, there is no use for male chicks born into this industry, so they are killed at birth, often through suffocation or being ground up alive and used as fertilizer (yes, you read that correctly). Female chicks are debeaked early on, which means that a portion of their beak is seared off without painkiller so that they don't peck their cagemates to death out of anxiety. The vast majority of egg-laying hens spend their lives in battery cages, which means that five to ten birds spend most of their lives in a space no bigger than the width of a standard sheet of paper. The relentless rubbing against the cages and standing on the wires results in severe damage to their little bodies—bodies that are forced to produce more than 250 eggs annually, compared to 100 eggs a century ago. At the end of their lives, when they are considered "spent," they are killed for low-grade meat.

Chickens Used for Meat

The vast majority of animals killed for food in the United States are birds—they make up roughly 99 percent of all the animals slaughtered. They are known as "broilers" by the industry, and have been bred to grow freakishly faster than they would in nature (the growth rate of a chicken is 300 percent greater than it was a half-century ago). The rapid growth of these birds often leads to acute heart failure once they've reached "market weight"; the chickens who survive are slaughtered at just forty-two days old and are oftentimes still peeping, not having yet learned to cluck (peeping is the sound baby birds make, similar to the *googoo-gaga* of human babies).

Turkeys

When we think of turkeys, many of us think of Thanksgiving or Christmas dinner, and leave it at that. We often don't consider the rest of the story, that just for the holiday season alone, 300 million turkeys are killed in the United States. They begin their lives by being hatched in a large incubator and after a few weeks are moved to giant, windowless sheds that they share with thousands of other turkeys, where they will spend the rest of their short lives (like other farmed animals, they are killed as babies—99 days for hens and 136 days for toms). A single worker could be caring for as many as thirty thousand birds, which of course often results in untreated illnesses and injuries. This kind of crowding causes the birds to injure one another with their sharp beak and toes, so—like chickens—they are debeaked using a hot blade, and it is also common for a portion of their toes to be removed with shears. The transport of these birds (and other farmed animals) is torture in and of itself—involving long distances as well as deprivation of water and food. Although the Humane Slaughter Act states that animals must be rendered insensible before they are shackled and slaughtered, the USDA does not interpret this law to include birds killed for food—including chicken and turkeys, who make up the vast majority of the animals killed for food in the United States. Therefore, there are virtually no laws that protect them (we will go over this further in Chapter 22).

Pigs

Although considered smarter than dogs, pigs are treated horrifically on factory farms. These outgoing, sensitive animals who (despite the stereotype) value cleanliness, spend their lives in cramped and filthy sheds. In the United States, mother pigs are often confined to gestation (prebirth) and farrowing (postbirth) crates that are so small that they can't turn around. They spend their lives repeatedly impregnated (which of course also means that hogs' semen is forcibly extracted) until they are considered "spent" and killed for their meat. Baby pigs are torn from their mother a few weeks after birth (the entire factory farming system is reliant on ripping families apart) and their bodies regularly undergo mutilations, including their tail being chopped off, the ends of their teeth being snipped with pliers, and males being castrated (no anesthesia, of course). When it is time for them to be transported to slaughter, while still babies at four to six months, the harsh weather conditions and long travels can result in them either overheating or freezing to death, depending upon the season and area (industry reports cite that more than a million pigs die in transport each year, with an additional forty thousand sustaining injuries by the time they reach the slaughterhouse). In light of the sheer number of pigs killed each year, improper stunning methods and throat-slitting result in many pigs still being conscious when they are dumped into large tanks of scalding water, which is intended to soften their skin and remove their hair.

Cows

Twenty-nine million cows are victims of the meat and dairy industries in the United States each year. Aside from the absolute horrors of the shamefully cruel dairy industry (which we detailed in Chapter

13), cows raised for meat are routinely branded with hot irons, dehorned (meaning their horns are gouged out, cut, or burned off), and castrated (males have their testicles ripped out of their scrotum). When they're big enough, beef cows are placed in dirty, outdoor feedlots. Ironically and tragically, cows raised for beef—who are killed at thirty-six months or younger—arguably have it the "best" in comparison to other animals who are part of the machine of factory farming. Cows raised for dairy, of course, are repeatedly impregnated (their babies are therefore repeatedly removed from them—the boys to become veal calves), and then, completely exhausted after four or so years, ultimately killed for low-grade beef.

Sheep and Goats

In the United States, sheep and goats are raised for their meat and milk, as well as for their fibers (Chapter 10 gets into that pretty deeply, as well as humane alternatives). Like pigs, they are tail-docked (to reduce the buildup of poop around their butt), which is either done by cutting it off without painkillers or by tying a rubber ring around it until it rots and falls off, which can lead to rectal prolapse and chronic pain. The wool production for a sheep declines with age, and when that happens, sheep are sent to slaughter. In Australia—which is where most of the world's wool comes from—these animals are frequently exported to Middle Eastern countries by sea, which can take weeks. Goats raised for meat are brutally slaughtered upon arrival, at just three to five months old.

Fish

Despite the convenient rumors, fish can indeed feel pain. And despite cultural catchphrases, they can have long memories (salmon can remember their homes after migrating thousands of miles) and are supersmart (goldfish can learn and remember skills). And yet aquaculture—the factory farming of aquatic animals—is one of the most rapidly growing sectors of animal-based food production. To date, humans eat more farmed fish than wild-caught (and by 2022, aquaculture output is predicted to rise by 33 percent). Nearly half of the fish consumed globally are raised in aquafarms where they live in cramped, dirty enclosures, are vulnerable to diseases, and regularly suffer injuries (frequently done to one another) and parasitic infections, all before being painfully slaughtered. And just because fish are wild-caught instead of farmed doesn't mean that things are okay; fishing is incredibly abusive in many ways. As one example, a terrible side effect from fishing is the tremendous amount of bycatch—these are nontarget animals who were basically at the wrong place at the wrong time (bycatch alone is estimated to be a ridiculous 8 percent of total catch—or 14 to 32 billion animals).

Okay, friend. You did it. You are officially through reading the hardest chapter of this book. Despite the disgusting horrors that point to a backward civilization that no feeling individual wants to be a part of, there are nonetheless some very bright lights worth noticing in the trajectory of food and social justice. First, it's very notable that a whopping 33 percent of Americans think animals should have the same protections as humans, which is up from 25 percent in 2008. That right there points to the fact that our collective value system does not match our collective behavior. When it comes to the harsh ways our society treats animals behind closed and locked doors, there is simply nowhere to go but up.

The complex-yet-simple issue of animal consumption is so deeply embedded in people's consciousness that it's really, really hard to break through—but it is indeed happening. Change for animals is occurring person by person, conversation by conversation, recipe by recipe, legislative bill by legislative bill, citywide resolution by citywide resolution, and revolutionary food product by revolutionary food product. To that end, thanks to the remarkable advent of cultured meat (which comes from the cell of an animal and does not require slaughter), the future of a meat-eating world is already written, and it's actually one we can all digest. The rest was just preamble. Now let's move on.

Personalities on the Farm

Farmed animals are not meat, dairy, and egg machines. When given the opportunity, they love to socialize, play, and dream, just like the companion animals we live with. All bacon once had a cute, wiggly tail, and that centerpiece turkey on the Thanksgiving table once had quite the social network.

HAPPY COWS

Cows are sensitive and emotional beings. They can pick up on stress experienced by another cow and also show learned fear responses to a person who has treated them roughly in the past. Mother cows also undergo extreme duress when their babies are taken away from them. A sign of a happy cow is one who likes to play and socialize, much like other animals, whether farmed or companion.

COURAGEOUS TURKEYS

If Benjamin Franklin had his way, the turkey would be United States' national bird instead of the eagle. He referred to them as "birds of courage," and seemed to admire these animals for their intelligence as well as curiosity. Turkeys are naturally social and playful animals and can recognize each others' voices.

COMMUNITY-MINDED CHICKENS

There is truth to the old "pecking order" adage, and it comes from chicken behavior. Chickens develop a social hierarchy within their communities, and they aren't shy about nipping another chicken if she steps out of line. When given free range—as opposed to being stuffed together in

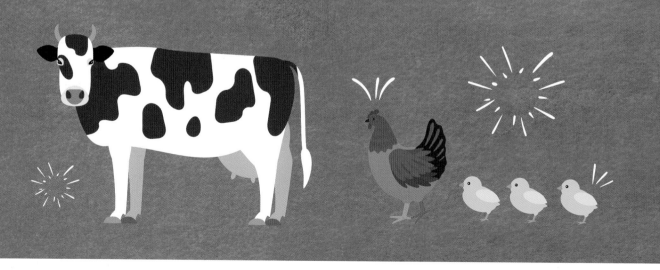

cages—adult chickens will teach young chickens important life skills, just as humans teach their youth the ways of the world.

PLAYFUL PIGGIES

While the right to live should not be based on a being's intelligence, we have to give pigs credit for their brainpower. Like dogs, pigs are extremely social and playful animals who love to romp and explore the world with their incredibly powerful sense of smell. Pigs also dream, respond when called by name, and can learn tricks.

ADVENTUROUS GOATS

There's a reason goat yoga is a thing; goats love to socialize! They are also inherently curious and like to climb, which is why you'll often find a goat precariously perched on a wooden beam or some other odd landing. If there's something to climb, you can bet on a goat to try it. Due to this curiosity, they're also adventurous foodies. A goat will try anything at least once, be that a new food or your brand-new vegan leather purse.

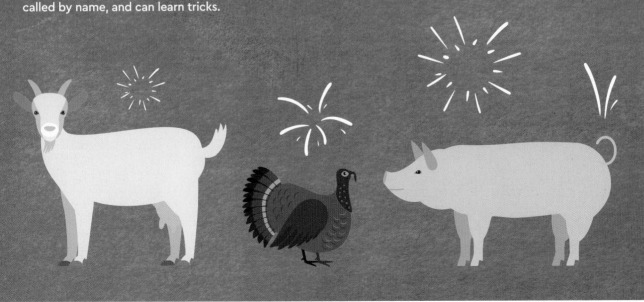

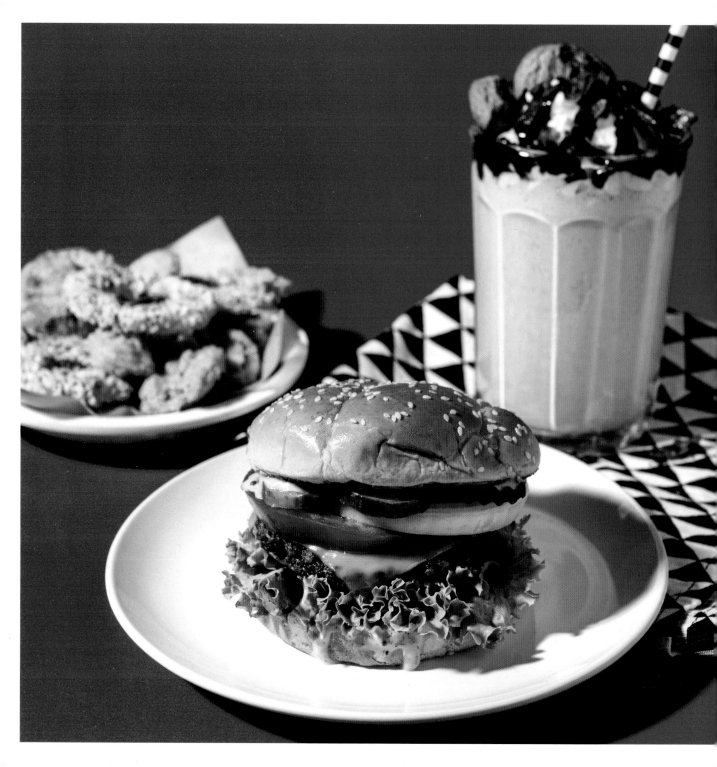

Classic Beefy Burger

Where's the beef? Right here! Only, these juicy patties are completely, deliciously animal-free. (Note: If "TVP granules" make you want to run to the nearest Burger King, just order the Impossible Whopper. Or grab a package of Beyond Burgers from the grocery store.)

¼ cup vegetable oil
3 cups sliced button mushrooms
1 tablespoon minced garlic
¾ cup vegan beef stock
1 cup small TVP (textured vegetable protein) granules

¼ cup nutritional yeast
½ cup vital wheat gluten
1 tablespoon dry mustard
1 tablespoon onion powder
¼ teaspoon freshly ground black pepper
¼ teaspoon liquid smoke

1 Preheat oven to 375°F and line a baking sheet with parchment paper. In a skillet over medium-high heat, heat 2 tablespoons of oil. Add mushrooms and garlic and sauté for 3 to 5 minutes, or until fragrant and mushrooms have reduced in size by about half. Add stock and bring to a simmer. Stir in TVP, cover, remove from heat, and let stand for 10 minutes.

2 Into a food processor, combine TVP mixture, nutritional yeast, vital wheat gluten, dry mustard, onion powder, pepper, and liquid smoke. Pulse a few times to mix, then process on low speed for about 1 minute, or until a dough ball forms.

3 Remove from food processor and divide into four equal portions. Form into patties and refrigerate for at least 20 minutes.

4 On baking sheet, place burgers in a single layer, cover tightly with foil, and bake for 20 minutes. Remove from oven.

5 In a skillet over medium-high heat, heat remaining 2 tablespoons of oil. Fry burgers for 2 minutes per side, or until a golden brown crust forms.

6 Serve with your favorite bun, cheese, and condiments.

A Pretty Easy Definition of "Humane"

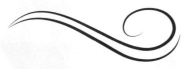

Day 21

"Humane" meat, milk, and eggs? ***Sorry, that's bullshit.***

You've learned

about the hideousness farmed animals go through in the factory farming industry, and maybe you're thinking, "What about animal products labeled 'humane'? Can I eat those?" After all, there's no shortage of signs in cute fonts that state the animals at such-and-such farm are treated better than the ones on big factory farms, with images of "happy" animals grazing on big expanses of land alongside choice words that undoubtedly allow believers to comfortably carry on with their omnivorous ways. And anyway, the meat inside that burger bun was locally produced. The cows' milk in that yogurt is organic. And the local café's scrambled eggs are from the owner's backyard flock where every chicken has a name. So, everything's cool, right? Not so fast.

Sadly, this inclination to continue to eat animals but to ensure they were treated "well" is self-deception at its best. Putting aside animals' innate will to live and indulging in a fantasy in which the animals don't suffer when they die, the systems of oppression that underlie animal agriculture simply cannot be avoided even when the animals are relatively well treated during their life. You can't have milk (even the organic variety) without taking babies away at birth, or very shortly thereafter—and regardless of whether that milk label is "non-GMO" or whatever, the boy offspring are ultimately raised for either veal or beef. No matter what. And you can't have egg-laying hens (even "free-range") without killing the boy chicks at birth; there is simply no place in the industry for the males. These examples of commodification are simply inherent in the industry of killing animals, even if someone slaps the word "happy" on the package.

If you are convinced that the cow or pig or goat body you are about to eat came from a scenario that's ethical because you spent a few extra dollars to ensure they had room to roam and you actually checked to make sure that the animals were being treated as advertised, consider this: the decision to eat an animal who came from a smaller operation where the animals had room to roam and not a giant factory farm might feel good on some level, but that feeling is rooted in a privilege that is our moral obligation to face. And it's this: *there is not enough land for everyone to eat animals raised that way*. Imagine if all Americans were to switch from consuming factory-farmed meat to meat from animals at small farms where they have more land, and you have suddenly created a system where the rich eat animals and the poor eat nothing. There is simply not enough land for this to be scalable.

But beyond the impasse created by a lack of land for these more "humanely" treated animals, there are also the issues of the labels themselves. Look deeper, and words like *cage-free*, *free-range*, and *grass-fed* do not carry the same gravitas you might hope for. The claims mislead customers to believe they are doing something that would comply with their ethical standards, but once you peel off that "humane" sticker, you can see that what goes on behind closed doors is anything but innocuous. Here's a little glossary:

Cage-free. Although cage-free systems purport to offer hens better lives than their caged sisters—and one could argue, on the surface, that this is marginally true—cage-free eggs are not all they're cracked up to be. This feel-good label can carry with it allowances such as no access to the outdoors, debeaking with no painkiller, and poor lighting in the sheds that can still house up to hundreds of thousands of birds. And the label has no bearing on what happens when these birds are sent to slaughter, so just like caged hens, cage-free hens are frequently transported long distances in crowded trucks—with no access to food or water—as they head to meet their fate. Hold onto your seatbelt, but, shockingly to many, the Twenty-Eight Hour Law—which states that animals can't be transported in confined cars for more than twenty-eight hours without stopping for rest, food, and water—*excludes all birds*.

Organic. There are some requirements that organic producers must allow animals to graze outside, but these conditions can vary greatly, and space allocations aren't clearly defined, leaving a lot of room for interpretation. The USDA standard is so lax that a commercial chicken farm can have a tiny screened-in concrete porch for thousands of chickens and still be labeled "organic."

Grass-fed. When you read that, do you think of a cow outside on vast pasture, munching on the grass and gazing placidly? Turns out that *grass-fed* only refers to what the animals *are fed*. So, a cow could be (and frequently is) fed hay in a feedlot on a factory farm and still be called grass-fed—and still can be subject to all that entails (including commonplace mutilations, such as dehorning, branding, and transport conditions).

There are, of course, a ton of labels—some of which mean more than others, and some of which mean basically nothing at all. There are also plenty of labels that don't require third-party certification, so basically, in these cases, there's zero auditing involved.

Humane. "Humane slaughter," the oxymoron to end all oxymorons. Notably, animals raised under many humane-sounding labels wind up at the same slaughterhouses as those who are factory-farmed. The vast majority of land animals killed for food in the United States (that's approximately 99 percent) are birds—and birds are actually excluded from the Humane Slaughter Act, which the USDA says "requires the proper treatment and humane handling of all food animals slaughtered in USDA-inspected slaughter plants," but goes on to say that "it does not apply to chickens or other birds." *What the?*

If you're *not* a bird, this "regulation" means that you should be stunned and rendered senseless before your throat is slit. Yet, we have all seen or at least heard about the many undercover investigations into slaughterhouses that show otherwise; animals who—due to the high-speed of these mechanized systems—are not successfully made unconscious before their throats are slit and they "bleed out," causing them tremendous suffering and a horrific death.

There are humane certification labels with stricter slaughter regulations that do include third-party auditing, and the animals who fall into these categories might wind up at smaller slaughterhouses. But even at smaller facilities that are compliant with the strictest humane labeling, the animals are still commodities—and can therefore experience the same problems of not being rendered unconscious before being killed. Incidents have been documented time and time again where the animal cries out in pain and fear as a second or third bolt is fired to his brain.

Kosher and halal. Many people assume that these animals are slaughtered more "humanely." This not true. In fact, in these instances, the law allows the animals to be fully conscious when their throats are slit in accordance with religious dictates.

Local. What about getting eggs from a backyard bird operation or the local farmers' market? First of all, it is very likely that the chicks themselves will have come from the same exact hatcheries as factory-farmed birds, where they never feel the love and protection of their factory-farmed mamas. In fact, they are hatched in incubators and then sent through the mail (yep, the good old US Postal Service), and—since boy chicks are unnecessary in the egg industry—on occasion, they are used as packing material to cushion the boxes.

There's also the simple reality of biology: Hens are only able to produce eggs for about half their lives. Since their full life span is around ten years, that means that unless you kill birds after they can't lay eggs anymore, you will eventually end up with a whole lot of chickens running around and eating feed, but not laying eggs.

But even in the most seemingly benign circumstance, you just can't escape the industry these birds came from, and the philosophical question of why we feel we "need" to use animal products at all is an important one here. The truth is, we don't need them, and they are not ours to take. If you want a chicken (and why wouldn't you? They can be great companions!), consider adopting a rescued one from a sanctuary, and providing them a lifelong home where they can just have the space to be their true, fabulous, authentic selves—which is, after all, pretty much what we're all seeking, isn't it?

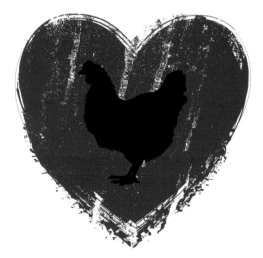

Animal Exploitation by the Numbers

According to extensive research by the Sentience Institute, factory farming in the United States is responsible for the vast majority of animals used for meat, milk, and eggs.

75%
The percentage of US adults who believe they usually eat meat, dairy, and eggs "from animals that are treated humanely"

99%
The percentage of farmed animals in the United States living in factory farms (including 74% of land animals and virtually all farmed fish)

- ❑ **70%** of cows
- ❑ **98%** of pigs
- ❑ **99%** of turkeys
- ❑ **98%** of chickens raised for eggs
- ❑ **99.9%** of chickens raised for meat

49%
The percentage of US adults that support a ban on factory farming

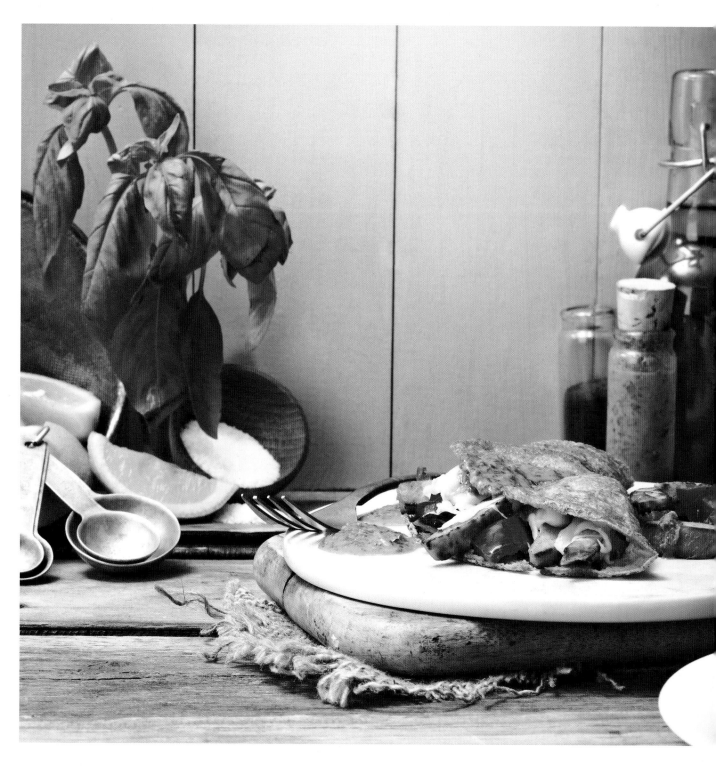

Lemon Pesto Omelet

Makes 2 omelets

Love eggy breakfasts but tired of the USDA's rampant corruption? This egg-free omelet will stick it to them.

Pesto:

1½	cups fresh spinach
1	cup fresh basil
⅓	cup fresh parsley
3	tablespoons olive oil
1	tablespoon lemon zest
3	tablespoons freshly squeezed lemon juice
3	garlic cloves, minced
1	teaspoon freshly ground black pepper
1	teaspoon nutritional yeast

Filling:

	Cooking spray for pan
¾	cup chopped vegan chicken
½	red bell pepper, seeded and diced
1	small zucchini, sliced
½	cup sliced mushrooms
½	cup vegan mozzarella cheese

Omelet:

1	(12-ounce) package firm tofu, drained and pressed
1	tablespoon unsweetened vegan milk
2	tablespoons nutritional yeast
1	tablespoon cornstarch
1½	teaspoons garlic powder
1	teaspoon Italian seasoning
¼	teaspoon ground turmeric
½	teaspoon freshly ground black salt
½	teaspoon paprika
2	tablespoons vegan butter

1 **Prepare the pesto:** In a food processor, combine all pesto ingredients and process until smooth. Cover and refrigerate.

2 **Prepare the filling:** Spray a cast-iron skillet with cooking spray and place over medium heat. Add chicken, bell pepper, zucchini, and mushrooms and cook until vegetables are tender. Transfer mixture to a medium-size bowl and cover.

3 **Prepare the omelet:** In a food processor, combine tofu, milk, nutritional yeast, cornstarch, garlic powder, Italian seasoning, turmeric, black pepper, salt, and paprika and process until smooth.

4 In a skillet over medium heat, melt 1 tablespoon of butter. Add half of omelet mixture, use a spatula to spread into a thin layer, and cook for 5 to 8 minutes. Once edges and underside begin to crisp, sprinkle ¼ cup of cheese over half of omelet, then top cheese with half of filling and ¼ cup of pesto. Cook until cheese begins to melt, then fold omelet over itself. Carefully slide omelet onto a serving plate and cover.

5 Repeat with remaining ingredients and serve omelets with remaining pesto drizzled over top.

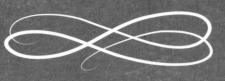

The USDA, Food Safety & Other Unicorns

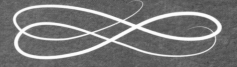

Day 22

*There's a pretty serious conflict of interest here, since the USDA oversees programs ("checkoff programs") that spend $557 million annually—money that is poured into advertising dollars and campaigns—**to encourage us to consume even more animal products**.*

The general

confidence in our modern government to protect us and the foods we eat is not singularly ruled by the noble intent to protect its people. Unfortunately, the government is equally interested in mollifying its lucrative industries and the powerful lobbyists that offer money and voting favors. The idea that the government regulates food with some kind of intact conscience is so entrenched in our belief system that we simply cannot believe that animals are treated as fleeting commodities with almost no laws governing their best interests.

Look deeper, and you'll find that the problem is more convoluted than it might have first seemed. In addition to the issues inherent in farmed animal law, meat and dairy products are heavily subsidized by the government. Fruit and vegetables, however, are barely subsidized at all to ensure they are afford-able and accessible. And yet the USDA's dietary food guidelines recommend that we fill up our plates with fruit, vegetables, grains, dairy, and protein (which can include meat, eggs, beans, peas, nuts, and seeds). Half of the plate on the dietary guidelines poster includes fruit and veggies.

According to the *Washington Post*, the federal food program was designed in hopes it "will lower obesity and such related illnesses as high blood pressure and cancer" since "animal fats contribute to these diseases and make up a larger percentage of the diet in America than in other countries." And even though the USDA dietary guidelines appear to be healthy, an entirely different reality is reflected when you look at the federal incentives to farmers. In a nutshell, the government pays farmers who grow food for animals who become meat.

The *Post* continues:

Of the roughly $200 billion spent to subsidize US commodity crops from 1995 to 2010 (commodity crops are interchangeable, storable foods, such as grains, certain beans, and cotton), roughly two-thirds went to animal-feed crops, tobacco, and cotton. Roughly $50 billion went to human-food crops, including wheat, peanuts, rice, oil seeds, and other crops that become sweeteners.

This policy started in the 1930s, when agricultural markets were suffering, particularly in the Midwest, and the proposed solution was to protect the national food supply by offering subsidies. But things evolve, and nowadays, healthy food advocates feel the policy should be dusted off and put in better alignment with the very guidelines that the USDA recommends.

Makes you wonder where the subsidies for fruit and vegetables are. Well, they are receiving just a small fraction of what goes into meat and dairy industries, which makes it no surprise that the USDA has shown that Americans consume fewer fruit and vegetables than ten years ago.

The meat of the matter is that our government uses "checkoff" programs to get us to buy more animal foods. Much like taxes, these programs are mandatory. According to the book *Meatonomics* by David Robinson Simon, it works like this: "Congress slaps a small assessment (less than 1 percent of wholesale price) on certain commodities, and the collected funds are used to pay for research and marketing programs that boost the sales."

So, when animal food producers collect $1 per head of cattle or 15¢ per 100 pounds of dairy, for example, they move those funds on to the marketers, and the proceeds are allocated among state and regional industry organizations throughout the country. It's these checkoff programs that in turn fund catchy slogans to get people to eat more meat ("Beef. It's What's for Dinner"; "Milk. It Does a Body Good"; and "The Incredible Edible Egg"). The USDA states that the investment return for each dollar of checkoff funds can yield as much as $18. Another way to look at it is that $557 million annually is generated for producers of animal foods so that they can promote their product.

This is our federal government at work. But if they stepped out—if the USDA ceased its involvement with checkoff programs that promote animal-based foods—the people who continue to get sick and die as a result of these foods might stand a fighting chance. So might the animals.

"Meatonomics" by the Numbers

In his book *Meatonomics: How the Rigged Economics of Meat and Dairy Make You Consume Too Much*, David Robinson Simon delves into the many forces behind the animal food system, including where it intersects with how and where we spend our money, and issues concerning our health. Here are some highlights of Simon's elaborate index of numbers that show the true economic cost of animal food.

$245: Average market value of a cow in the North Central United States

$498: Average cost to raise a cow in that region

$38 billion: Amount US taxpayers spend annually to subsidize meat and dairy

$17 million: Amount US taxpayers spend annually to subsidize fruit and vegetables

$557 million: Amount the US government spends annually on "checkoff programs" to promote meat and dairy

$51 million: Amount the US government spends annually to promote fruit and vegetables

33%: Percentage of US cancer, diabetes, and heart disease cases related to meat and dairy consumption

0: Dietary cholesterol needed by humans according to the National Academies' Institute of Medicine

300 milligrams: Daily maximum recommended dietary cholesterol, per USDA

25%: Average percentage by which a vegan's blood cholesterol level is lower than an omnivore's

18%: Average percentage by which by which a vegan's weight is lower than an omnivore's

172,000: Human lives that a 50% excise tax on meat and dairy would save yearly

26 billion: Animal lives that a 50% excise tax on meat and dairy would save yearly

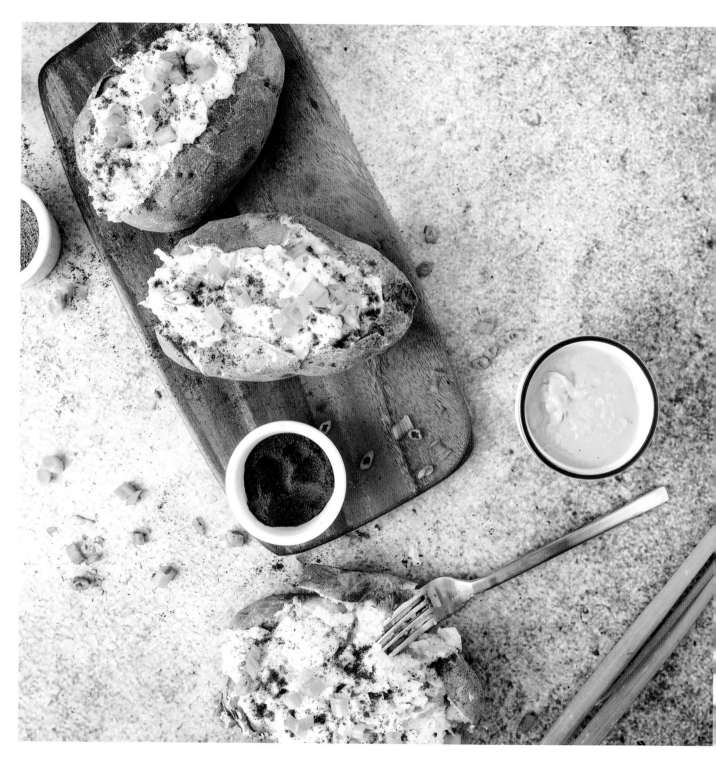

Deviled Egg Baked Potatoes

Serves 2

Just because you're cutting eggs from your diet doesn't mean you can't enjoy classic eggy flavors. Turn everyone's favorite party appetizer into a totally vegan main with the help of potatoes!

2   large russet potatoes, scrubbed
⅓   cup unsweetened plain soy milk
¼   cup vegan mayonnaise
2   tablespoons yellow mustard
1   teaspoon seasoned salt

1   teaspoon dried dill
½   teaspoon granulated onion
⅛   teaspoon freshly ground black pepper
2   tablespoons sliced scallions, for garnish
Paprika, for garnish

❶ Preheat oven to 350°F. Bake potatoes directly on rack for 1 hour, or until tender. Remove from oven and let cool until able to handle.

❷ Slice open top of potatoes and scoop out flesh into a small bowl. To bowl, add soy milk, mayonnaise, mustard, salt, dill, onion, and pepper. Mix well until smooth, adding 1 tablespoon more soy milk if too dry. Stuff filling into potato skins, sprinkle with scallions and paprika, and serve immediately.

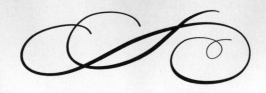

It's Your Party. Drink Wine If You Want To!

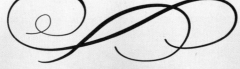

Day 23

*If you heard wine and beer aren't vegan, you heard wrong. So, **pour yourself a glass of vegan pinot while you read this chapter.***

First, the ugly:

it's true that some wine uses fining agents during production—namely through (wait for it . . .) fish bladders (similar to the filtering of sugar through bone char).

Fining is a clarification process used to remove unwanted particles in wine that could affect its overall color, taste, or aroma. This process results in a wine that is considered by some to be "cleaner." In addition to the fish bladders (more specifically, isinglass—or gelatin from fish bladder membranes), some wineries also use egg whites, bone marrow, gelatin, casein (milk protein), blood, and chitin (fiber from crustacean shells) for the fining process. Now, the good news: vegan alternatives to these animal-derived agents do exist, including carbon, bentonite clay, limestone, plant casein, silica gel, and vegetable plaques.

Even better, many of your favorite alcoholic libations are probably vegan, and there are really easy ways to find out. Barnivore.com (there's an app, too) is about to be your new drinking buddy. It has an extensive, searchable database where you can type in the name of the boozy beverage (be it wine, beer, or spirits) you're contemplating purchasing and find out whether it passes the vegan test. Many do (including the red variety of surprisingly adequate three-buck Chuck at Trader Joe's, so cheers to that!). Another tip-off: the words "unfined and unfiltered" on the label mean that it very likely is vegan.

You may be wondering about biodynamic wines. Although these wines are often pricier and fancier—and they employ more sustainable production systems—many of these types of wines involve animal exploitation, sadly. The winemaking process itself used at these vineyards is indeed vegan (a grape is a grape is a grape), but the growing practices frequently are not. Biodynamic wine follows a practice of agriculture that relies on both scientific and spiritual elements (called anthroposophy), but since this type of wine is organic, the production not only relies on animal manure, but also sometimes pieces of dead animals (which help to incubate the poop)—this might include cow skulls, horns, and intestines. *Blech.*

Can biodynamic wine be made vegan? The short answer is yes, but finding vegan biodynamic vineyards is still uncommon. One example of a company that's both biodynamic and vegan is Querciabella, which rigorously avoids all animal products. This forward-thinking company uses "green manure" (which comes from composted plants instead of animal poop). Querciabella even grows its own herbs (for the compounds it sprays) and seeds for cover-crop mixes.

So, you see, anything can be done without animal exploitation—even vegan biodynamic wine (not that you need biodynamic wine to enjoy a glass of vino after a tough week). And if you're more of a beer person, opt for Guinness, Budweiser, Miller Lite, Heineken, or—for the hipsters—Pabst.

And what about that bar on the corner where you and your friends have beers after work? Or the cute little restaurant where you go specifically because of its bottomless Sunday brunch mimosas? How do you know if they are vegan? It might be overwhelming to think that in addition to changing your food, you now need to pay attention to things like fining agents in wine, too.

Here's the thing: don't. Don't pay attention to it. At least not for now. As we've said before, don't let the perfect be the enemy of the good—especially in your early days of living on the plant-side. Many vegans (new and seasoned alike) make sure that any wine or beer bottles they buy *for home* are cruelty-free, but they take a somewhat more liberal approach when they are, say, at that bar. In other words, when out and about, they don't check to see whether the alcohol at the pub involved animal-derived filtering agents or production methods. That might be a route you choose, too.

Some vegans also take on the added responsibility of feeling they should present their new lifestyle as low-maintenance to make their friends see it as accessible and not limiting. Not nit-picking all the time has that added value, too; we can scour labels for hidden animal products all we want when we're at the grocery store, but perhaps the pub isn't the best place to aim for perfection. Do what you can, and drink what you want (*responsibly* . . . which also means taking a Lyft home).

Stop Whining

Vegans can have their wine and hangover, too.

In addition to the plethora of cruelty-free beers and wines you'll find at Barnivore.com—not to mention at your local liquor store—here are some compassionate companies that sell their vegan wine online. We'll drink to that!

- China Bend Winery
- Cooper's Hawk Vineyards
- Fitzpatrick Winery
- Palmina Wines
- Querciabella
- Smithfield Wine
- Thumbprint Cellars
- The Vegan Vine Wines
- Vinavanti Wines
- Wrights Wines

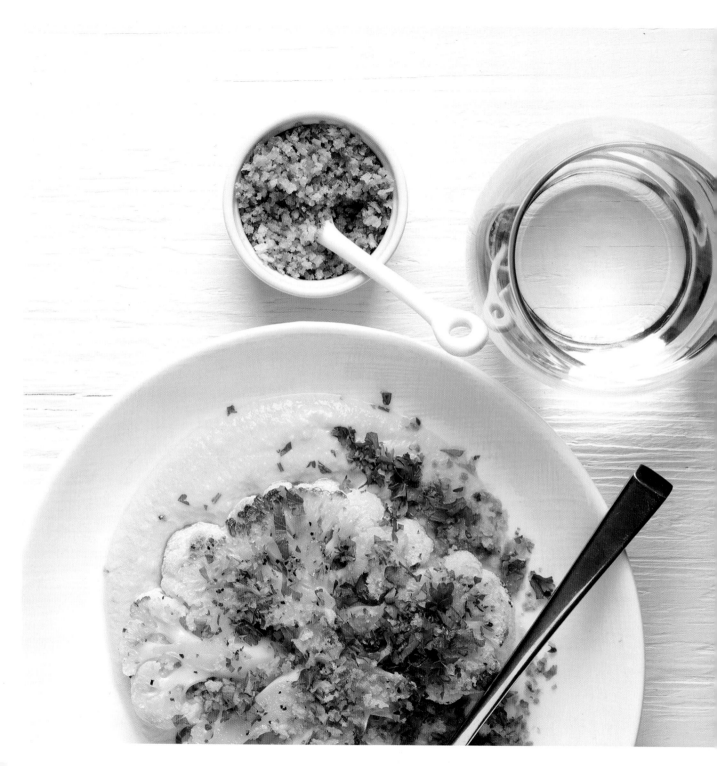

Roasted Cauliflower Steaks
with White Wine Cream Sauce

Serves 4

Pair this satiating and sophisticated dish with a vegan red wine, and you have the makings for a totally romantic, plant-based dinner.

Cooking spray, for pan

Cauliflower steaks:

1	large head cauliflower
1½	tablespoons olive oil
⅛	teaspoon salt
⅛	teaspoon freshly ground black pepper

Cream sauce:

2¼	cups water
¾	cup white wine
⅔	cup raw, unsalted cashews, soaked in water for 2 hours, then drained (if you don't have 2 hours, cover the cashews with boiling water and soak for 20 minutes, then drain)
4	garlic cloves, minced
¼	cup nutritional yeast
2	teaspoons fine sea salt
¼	cup minced fresh parsley, for garnish

1 Preheat oven to 425°F. Line a baking sheet with parchment paper and coat with cooking spray.

2 **Prepare the cauliflower:** Remove leaves and carefully trim stem, leaving core intact. Using a large knife, cut cauliflower from top to bottom into four ¾-inch-thick steaks. Lightly brush one side of cauliflower steaks with oil and sprinkle with salt and pepper. Place on prepared baking sheet and roast in the oven for 30 minutes, or until golden brown.

3 While cauliflower is roasting, prepare the white wine cream sauce: In a blender, combine water, wine, soaked cashews, garlic, nutritional yeast, and salt and blend until smooth and creamy. Transfer sauce mixture to a saucepan and cook over medium-high heat for 5 minutes, stirring as needed, until reduced to the consistency of thick cream.

4 To serve, pour ½ cup sauce onto a plate and place one roasted cauliflower steak on top. Sprinkle with 1 tablespoon of parsley. Repeat with remaining cauliflower steaks and serve immediately.

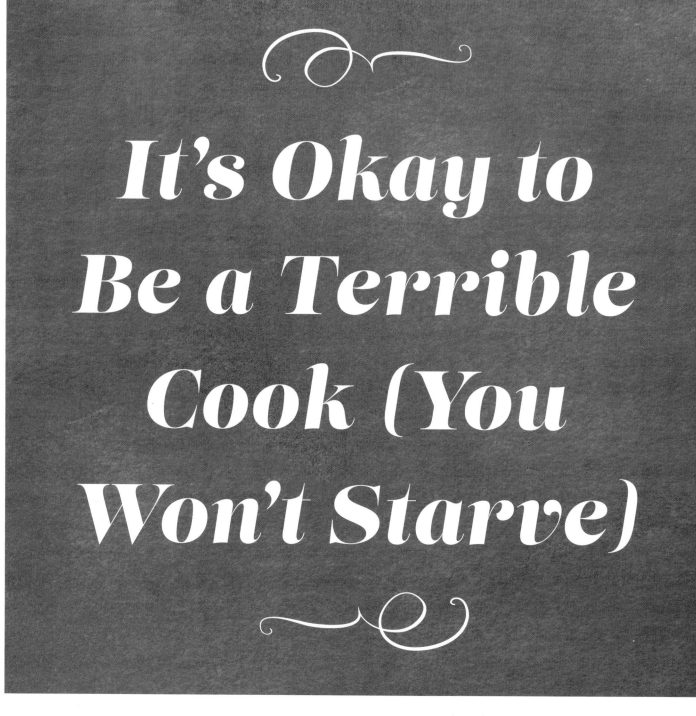

Day 24

You don't have to be a good cook to be vegan, just as you don't have to be a good cook to be not vegan.

It's pretty

simple: if you so choose, you can just stick with exactly the same foods you used to eat before you went plant-based and stick to making the vegan equivalent of those (because #thereisaveganversionofeverything).

You'll find that more often than not, just a few simple swaps will veganize your meal. The spices you use are almost definitely already vegan (but all you really need is garlic salt anyway), and many of the sauces are too (if they're not, making them vegan will be a supersimple switch or introduction to a new product at your store). Your pasta with meat sauce can become pasta with marinara and Beyond Meat sauce. The weeknight stir-fry? Swap out the fish sauce for Trader Joe's Soyaki Sauce and use tofu or vegan meat instead of chicken. There are even vegan hot pockets and a plethora of frozen dinners,

if that's your definition of "cooking" (no judgment). And let's not forget the "I'm-an-adult-and-can-eat-what-I-want-so-I'm-having-cereal-for-dinner" meal. That's usually already vegan, as long as you fill your bowl with almond, soy, coconut, cashew, hemp, oat (you get the picture) milk, and make sure your cereal has no animal products lurking in there.

But even if you don't fancy yourself a cook, going vegan could very well inspire you to try your hand at it. That doesn't mean that you would be doing it because you have to; rather, some people find a lot of inspiration from the new foods, cuisines, ingredients, and taste profiles they are suddenly discovering, and they find that their inner–Julia Child is dying to emerge. If that's you, huzzah! But do be patient with yourself. You might choose to start off with a few simple cookbooks, including *Veganomicon* by Isa Chandra Moskowitz and Terry

Hope Romero, *The Vegan Planet* by Robin Robertson, *Vegan Comfort Classics* by Lauren Toyota, and *Simple Happy Kitchen* by Miki Mottes.

Finally, don't knock ordering in. City-dwellers all over have gotten quite accustomed to it, and—assuming you live in a place that offers delivery—it can seriously rock your world. Many Chinese places offer dishes with bean curd (which is just tofu, a staple in Asian cuisine), and there are few better items than fried bean curd with broccoli and brown rice (frequently, the fortune cookies are also vegan, but do check the ingredients). Beyond Chinese, more and more midsize to large cities also boast vegan-friendly pizza as well as Thai food (just make sure there's no fish sauce). Download the Happy Cow app so that you can immediately pinpoint vegan-friendly restaurants no matter where you are; use the search functions on such sites as Yelp, Grubhub, or Postmates to choose vegetarian or vegan; and frequent Asian or Mexican spots, which are way more likely than classic American joints to offer vegan meals (if you do go for Mexican, you can almost always rely on a solid burrito full of beans, rice, salsa, lettuce, and guac—just confirm they don't cook the beans or rice in lard, or that they add cheese). One last thing: if you do order in, remember to tip well—never below 20 percent! In other words, don't be a cheapskate.

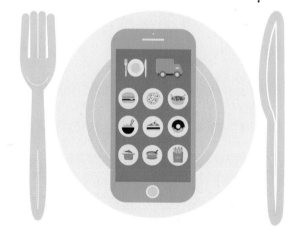

Build a Bowl

One of the most simple-to-make, satisfying-to-eat, and impressive-to-post dishes is a scrumptious and satiating bowl. Here's how you do it.

1 START WITH A BASE

This should be your favorite cooked grain (brown rice, quinoa, millet, amaranth, or polenta), potato (cooked however you like best), cauliflower rice, zoodles, or noodles.

2 NEXT UP COMES YOUR FAVORITE GREEN

Go for steamed kale, spinach, collards (remember that those take longer to cook than most other greens), spring mix, romaine, or any combination of the above.

3 ADD YOUR PROTEIN OF CHOICE

Obviously, we all know by now that greens and grains also have protein, but step it up and make it a more filling dish by adding tofu, tempeh, seitan, or your favorite meat analogue that is a great add-on in a bowl. Do a quick sauté or crispify your protein in an air-fryer (and hey, a microwave works too).

4 CONSIDER BEANS

For even more added protein, texture, and rich layers of taste, add in your favorite bean (such as chickpeas—even if they're straight from the can, we won't tell) or edamame.

5 KEEP IT SAUCY

The final (and possibly most important) step in your perfect bowl is to top it off with your favorite sauce. Tahini is always an easy option and is loaded with good-for-you fat that will keep you full and happy for a long time, but you can also whip up a tangy peanut sauce in your blender by thinning out some peanut butter with a little water, adding in a few simple spices, and perhaps tossing in just a tiny bit of hot sauce for a kick. If you're feeling adventurous, sprinkle the bowl with nutritional yeast (affectionately known among seasoned vegans as "nooch"), garlic salt, and sesame seeds.

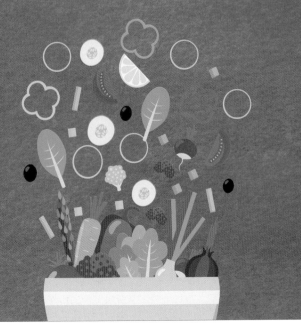

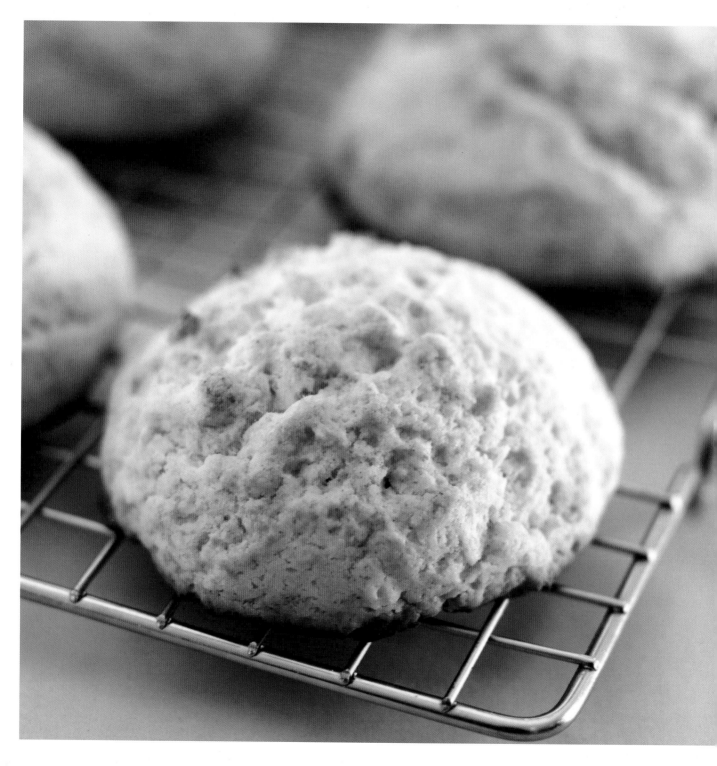

Two-Step Biscuits

Makes 12 biscuits

These cheesy biscuits taste great out of the oven or smothered with your favorite gravy.

1	cup unsweetened vegan milk
2	tablespoons lemon juice
2¼	cups all-purpose flour
¼	cup nutritional yeast
2	tablespoons sugar
2	teaspoons baking powder
1	teaspoon baking soda
1½	teaspoons salt
¼	cup refined coconut oil, chilled until solid
½	cup finely chopped chives

1 Preheat oven to 450 degrees. Line a baking sheet with parchment paper or Silpat. In a small bowl, mix milk and lemon juice. Set aside. In a large bowl, mix flour, nutritional yeast, sugar, baking powder, baking soda, and salt. Using a pastry cutter or your fingers, work chilled coconut oil into flour until it resembles fine crumbs. Create a well in center of dough and add milk and lemon juice mixture. Mix gently, and sprinkle in chives. Gently knead until it comes together.

2 On a well-floured surface, form dough into a ¾-inch-thick rectangle. Using a 2-inch round cookie cutter, cut out 12 biscuits. Gently reform dough as necessary to make all biscuits, being careful not to over-knead. Transfer biscuits to baking sheet, and bake for 10 to 12 minutes or until lightly browned. Remove from oven and let rest for 5 minutes before serving.

Self–Righteousness Is for Losers

Day 25

*The fact that the purchasing power of vegans is in direct contrast with societal norms and therefore shakes things up **doesn't mean vegans are self-righteous** (even though some definitely are).*

Vegans can

sometimes get a really bad rap when it comes to the idea that we're always rolling our eyes, always judging the person in front of us at the café who puts cows' milk in their coffee, or making very clear that *we are better than everyone else*. And the fact is, some people—vegan and not—are just assholes. After all, #thereisaveganversionofeverything. #ohmygodstopsayingit.

As you can probably tell, a lot of vegans are very passionate—especially those who are in it for the animals. Many of us feel that when we learned what was going on behind closed doors for animals, a veil lifted. Over time, many vegans become strong communicators about their choice to not eat or use animal products—remembering that we are each on our journeys, everyone is

different, and nobody goes vegan by being shamed into it.

But we didn't necessarily all have that kind of decorum at the beginning. That "how could I not have known?" question haunts a lot of us, so some of us turn it around to others, which understandably comes off as self-righteous despite the good intentions. Of course, intentions don't erase bad communication skills—hence the perception that vegans are self-righteous. But it does at least put that "self-righteousness" somewhat into context.

As for annoying vegans, here's the thing: they were almost certainly annoying before they went vegan. While going vegan does not mean they need to sit on a moral high ground (since really, nobody should sit on a moral high ground), the more that veganism grows in popularity, the more likely it is that our movement will have a few (or more than a few) folks who are smug and sanctimonious. On the flip side though, the bigger veganism becomes, the more it will also attract expert communicators, kind and thoughtful do-gooders, and all-around humble folks who are doing their best to live authentically while also being respectful and approachable. And that latter category fits the bill for most of the vegans you will meet—we'll bet the farm (sanctuary) on that.

For some, going vegan means adopting a whole new worldview. We used to think eating animals was justifiable behavior. Either that, or we just didn't think about it at all. Once we started to think about our choices with a bit more self-honesty, most of us felt walloped. We had to look at our previous behavior with a new kind of discernment that is seriously uncomfortable to face. Learning about what farmed animals endure can create a kind of PTSD for some people, so in a way, it makes sense that new vegans who are bearing witness to animal cruelty find themselves frustrated with those who don't want to give up their bacon. Again, this is usually ironed out in time, and longtime vegans find ways of coping with the reality of living in a meat-eating world while still enjoying their life.

Just as we're not all self-righteous, neither are we a bunch of sad sacks crying our eyeballs out and thinking about death all the time. Many who stop eating animals do so because they have a firm resolution to show up better for themselves and for the world. That relentless self-examination often coexists with a deep empathy toward all beings and a refusal to be complacent.

Compassion is the through-line here—whether we're talking about animals or people. Its synonyms include mercy, kindness, and empathy. Just as so many of us go vegan because we can't stomach taking part in a system that is at its core so heartless to animals, the same can be said about extending compassion to other humans . . . even if they aren't vegan.

One surefire way to not be an asshole is to relentlessly stay in gratitude. If we focus on the animals whom we have saved instead of putting all of our energy, all the time, into the ones who weren't—because of our former omnivorous ways, or because the person in front of us is eating a piece of bacon while laughing at our delicious seitan drumstick—we will not do anyone any good (not the animals, and not ourselves). We've got to be in it for the long run, and sometimes, that means we have to stop fighting the person in front of us (who is probably, *ahem*, self-righteous) who might not be ready to go vegan yet. We don't need to always have the last word.

Finally, it's superimportant to have safe spaces in which to air your frustrations. That way, you have a place to put it all—especially during those times when you refuse to take the bait, because you're a fabulous human doing fabulous work in this world, showing up as fabulously as you can, and you don't have to hold on your fabulous shoulders the not-so-fabulous weight of the world.

How Not to Be a Self-Righteous Asshole (Vegan or Otherwise)

Ever wonder whether you're appearing holier-than-thou? Here are some basic dos and don'ts for communicating like a pro (and preserving your sanity, while you're at it).

DO: Consider your audience. If you are talking to your combative brother who considers it his duty in this world to always take the opposite perspective of whatever you say, then he's not the right person to hand a vegan leaflet to while he's eating a piece of steak.

DON'T: Be a doormat. Just because your brother is a jerk doesn't mean you have to take abuse. You can always be gracious, you can choose to not take his bait, you can walk away, and you can also explain how it's not okay to be mean to you.

DO: Take it easy on yourself *and* on others. You don't always have to be the spokesperson for veganism, and the person you're trying to reach with your message doesn't have to get it the first time. Be gracious.

DON'T: Scream at people (whether that means people on the street buying a hot dog, your roommate who just bought a new wool sweater, or your mom who stuffed your stocking with makeup that isn't cruelty-free).

DO: Enjoy yourself. Your veganism is the best part of you. Don't let anyone else take that from you or dim your light.

DON'T: Take every little thing too seriously. Life is short, and not everything warrants a big to-do. This doesn't mean you're self-abandoning; it means you're respecting your energy and bandwidth.

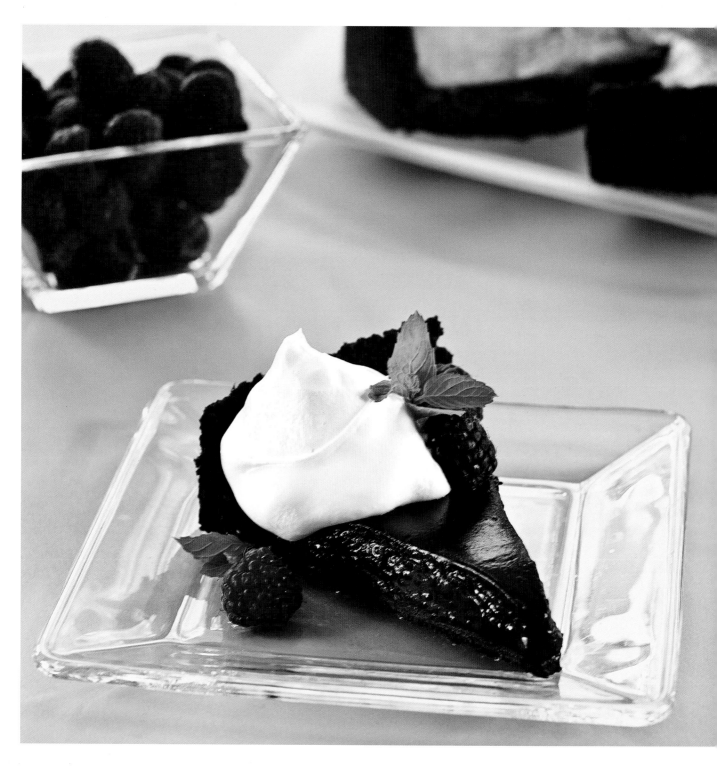

Heavenly Dark Chocolate Torte

Exquisitely silky and rich, this truffle-inspired dessert nestled in a chocolate shortbread crust is simply better than all other desserts.

Crust:
¾ cup brown rice flour
⅔ cup almond meal
⅔ cup cane sugar
½ cup unsweetened cocoa powder
¼ cup arrowroot powder
½ cup vegan butter

Filling:
1¼ cups vegan creamer
1½ cups chocolate chips
1 (3-ounce) vegan dark chocolate bar, roughly chopped
2 teaspoons pure vanilla extract
Vegan whipped cream, for topping
Raspberries, for topping

❶ **Prepare the crust:** Preheat oven to 350°F. In a medium-size bowl, whisk together flour, almond meal, sugar, cocoa powder, and arrowroot powder. Add vegan butter and stir well to form a soft dough. Press dough 1 inch deep into bottom and sides of an ungreased 9-inch tart pan with a removable bottom. Bake for 12 to 14 minutes, or until slightly puffed. Remove from oven and allow to cool completely on a wire rack, then remove outer ring.

❷ **Prepare the filling:** In a saucepan over medium heat, bring vegan creamer to a boil. Remove from heat. Add remaining ingredients; stir until chocolate is melted and mixture is smooth. Cover and chill in refrigerator for 15 minutes.

❸ Pour filling into prepared crust and chill for 1 hour, or until firm. Garnish outer edge of torte with vegan whipped cream and raspberries.

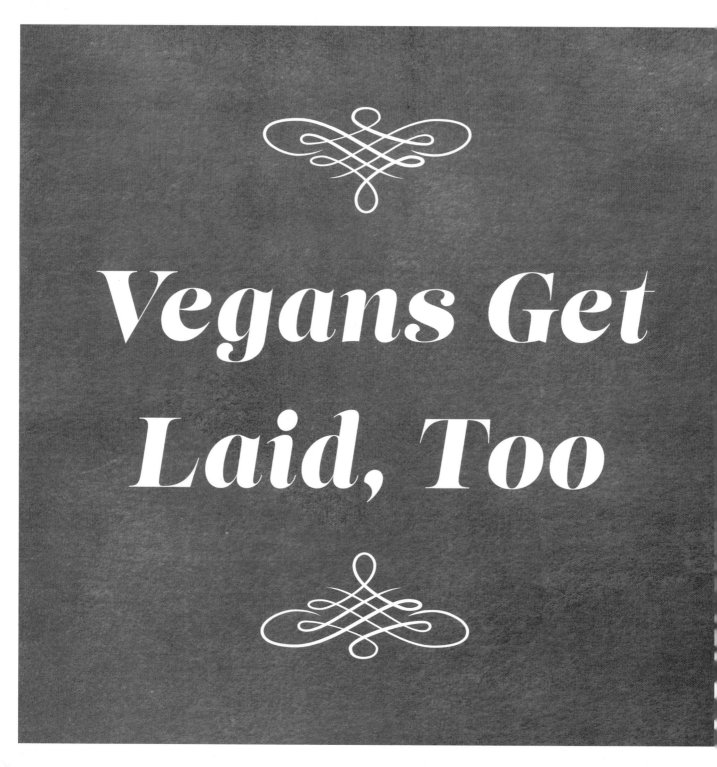

Vegans Get Laid, Too

Day 26

Everyone all at once: We do! ***And it's better!***

And now for

the real point of this book: vegans have better sex. It's true, trust us. A vegan diet has a slew of benefits for our health—which you've probably already picked up if you're reading this front to back—and that includes our sexual health and the health of our reproductive organs.

Let's talk about penises, shall we? Because every good book about veganism should, at some point, talk about penises. Frighteningly, erectile dysfunction affects up to thirty million people in the United States. When arteries clog, it can result in decreased blood flow to the penis (as well as to the brain and heart)—which can be a common issue that happens when we eat animal products. On the flip side, a whole foods-based vegan diet can actually reduce the buildup of plaque in the arteries, allowing blood to flow freely, helping to improve sexual health. The

Journal of the American Medical Association came out with a study stating that nearly one-third of participants experienced a return to normal of their sexual function by lowering the amount of saturated fat and cholesterol they were consuming and upping their fiber. *Cough cough GO VEGAN cough cough.*

In addition to better blood flow, eating plant-based means you taste better. A study in *Chemical Senses Journal* found that men who eat vegan meals packed with fruit and vegetables have sweeter-tasting semen (yes, there is actual science behind that old "pineapple juice" trick). *Cough cough GO VEGAN cough cough* (ugh, this cough!).

That same study found that people who eat plant-based smelled significantly better than meat-eaters. Why? One reason might be that consuming red meat results in the release of toxins into the bloodstream and large intestines, eventually making it out through our pores (yes, meat stink). There's also the fact that the bacteria on our skin can thrive on meat-eaters—since bacteria consume fats and proteins, which meat contains in spades.

Moving on. Let's now talk about vaginas. According to gynecologist (and longtime vegan) Stacy De-Lin, MD, when it comes to vaginal health, probiotic-rich foods are your best friend. As she told VegNews, "Nondairy yogurt and kefir are chock-full of healthful probiotics and the bacteria lactobacillus, both which help to keep your vagina at a healthy pH level and fend off yeast and excess bacteria," she says. Anyone else suddenly feeling the urge to eat a vegan Greek yogurt parfait?

Then there's the benefits of soy (which we cover in detail in Chapter 16). Of the many advantages of this wonder food, one is its connection to sexual health. Got a vagina? Think of soy as a natural lube from the inside out. Got a pecker? Soy isoflavones are proven to be great for prostate health; without a healthy prostate gland, libido would decline, along with fertility and hormone balance.

Once your reproductive organs are healthy, chances are, you're going to want to do it ("Alexa: play 'Let's Get It On'"). Dr. De-Lin recommends regular STD testing, adding that the most effective way to prevent STDs is through using condoms—but you're going to want to make sure that your enjoyment is not at the behest of anyone else's torture. In other words, make sure those condoms are vegan. "While some condoms are processed with the milk protein casein, plenty of safe and effective vegan brands exist, like paraben-free Glyde, fair-trade and hypoallergenic Sustain, all-natural Sir Richard's, and the allergen-friendly, latex-free Unique Plus," De-Lin tells us. These brands are available wherever you get your condoms, as well as online. So, pick your favorite and start stocking your glove compartment, nightstand, pockets, and purses.

If a fabulous sex life is a priority for you—and why wouldn't it be?—then you have ever more reason to ditch animal products and go vegan. Be careful out there, lover; you're about to become even more desirable than you already were . . . as if that were even possible.

5 Foods to Get You in the Mood

We all know that what you eat influences your health in powerful ways. But did you know food can play a major role in your sex life as well? Foods high in the amino acid L-arginine, for example, are known to increase nitric oxide, which in turn dilates arteries and blood vessels to improve blood flow to all the right places. Here are five super-sources of L-arginine that'll turn the heat up and get your blood pumping in no time.

PUMPKIN SEEDS	7 grams per cup	These nutty seeds are one of the richest sources of L-arginine. Try them roasted and sprinkled over your salad at lunch to turn up the romance after dinner.
SOYBEANS	5.8 grams per cup	Good news—these protein-rich legumes will also help get things steamy in the bedroom, so throw a few cubes of tofu into your stir-fries, soups, and smoothies. Your partner will thank you.
NORI	4.6 grams per cup	Who knew this underwater weed was such a powerhouse? In addition to its blood-pumping properties, it helps release hormones for libido and a more youthful appearance.
WALNUTS	4.5 grams per cup	Bake up a batch of vegan chocolate chip cookies as a romantic gesture for your sweetheart, and seal the deal by sprinkling in some L-arginine-loaded walnuts into the batter.
CHICKPEAS	3.8 grams per cup	These Middle Eastern marvels are the embodiment of versatility. Not only can you use them to turn up the heat in your sex life, but you can heat things up by using them in buffalo chickpea tacos. Win-win!

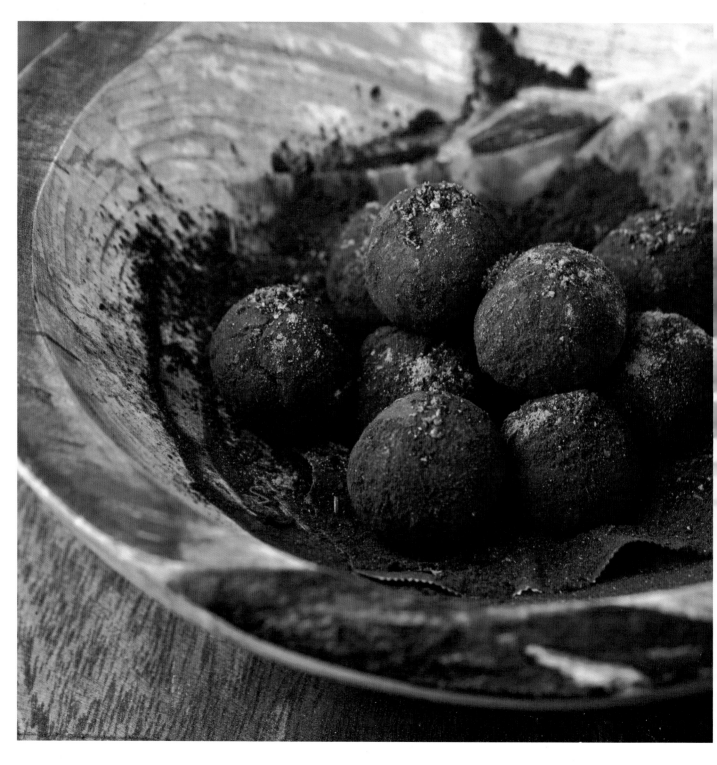

Chocolate Chile Truffles

Turn up the heat with these sensuously sweet-and-spicy chocolate treats, kicked up a notch with ancho chile and cinnamon.

8 ounces vegan dark chocolate, finely chopped	¼ teaspoon salt
¾ cup unsweetened vegan milk	2 teaspoons olive oil
2 tablespoons coconut sugar	½ teaspoon pure vanilla extract
2 teaspoons ancho chile powder	¼ cup unsweetened cocoa powder, sifted
½ teaspoon ground cinnamon	

1 Place chocolate in a heatproof bowl. In a small saucepan over medium heat, combine vegan milk, coconut sugar, 1½ teaspoons ancho chile powder, cinnamon, and ⅛ teaspoon salt. Bring to a low boil, whisking continuously. Remove from heat and allow milk mixture to sit for 30 minutes, whisking occasionally.

2 Return saucepan to heat and bring milk mixture to a low boil again. Remove from heat and immediately pour milk through a fine-mesh strainer over chocolate, completely covering it. Cover bowl and let sit undisturbed 4 minutes.

3 Add olive oil and vanilla and whisk, from center out, to form a smooth and glossy ganache. Pour into a shallow dish and let cool at room temperature for 30 minutes. Refrigerate, uncovered, until surface is no longer soft, then place parchment paper directly onto ganache, covering completely, and refrigerate for at least 3 hours, until very firm.

4 Remove from refrigerator. Using a teaspoon, scoop out 1-inch portions, rolling and shaping into balls (if ganache becomes too soft to shape, refrigerate until cold and continue). Cover and refrigerate truffles for 25 minutes.

5 In a small bowl, whisk together cocoa powder, remaining ½ teaspoon of ancho chile powder, and remaining ⅛ teaspoon of salt. Roll truffles in mixture, coating evenly, and serve at room temperature.

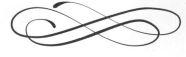

You Can Be Vegan and Travel and Not Die!

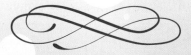

Day 27

*Like every single other aspect of traveling, being vegan on the road just requires some really simple planning . . . **but it's not hard**.*

A portion of this book was written on a cross-country Amtrak trip from Chicago to Los Angeles, choo-chooing straight through America's heartland: Illinois, Kansas, Colorado, New Mexico, Arizona. You may not think of train travel as having the best vegan options (you may not think of train travel as an option at all, but we'll get to planes and automobiles soon, don't worry), but Amtrak offers a vegan breakfast, lunch, and dinner item, including a rigatoni with soy sausage and a pretty darn good veggie burger—not to mention soy milk for the coffee, no extra charge. These menu staples point to an important sign of the times: there is vegan food everywhere.

Whether you're flying around the world or road-tripping to the top of the state, trust us: as a vegan-on-the-road, you will not starve. That doesn't mean there won't be times when you'll need to specifically seek it out, going that extra mile (sometimes literally) to ensure you have vegan schmear for your bagel. Sure, there will be moments when you'll find yourself at a nonveg restaurant and you'll need to have them "hold the cheese and mayo" or switch out the egg for an avocado in that sandwich, but asking for these simple swaps—and reading menus with an eye toward what-could-be—will eventually become old hat for you. And with more and more fast-food restaurants offering vegan options (check out our mouthwatering list in Chapter 6), your traveling days as a new vegan will be easy-peasy.

If you're newly veg and are nervous about food for your upcoming trip, know this: you will eat well, you will not go hungry, and your veganism will add a meaningful and fun layer to your travels. If you're going with another vegan, or with someone who is supportive of you and is veg-curious, then you two will have a fun time gallivanting around the vegan-friendly options found on the Happy Cow app, or (for international travelers) using the superhelpful app Veganagogo to locate nearby restaurants while concurrently translating important vegan-related turns of phrase to the local language (such as "I am vegan" with a description of what that means and a request for the server to point to the items on the menu that do not include animal products). Other helpful apps for traveling include AirVegan, which tells you where you can get plant-based food in airport terminals around the globe; and VeganXPress, which will help you find vegan options at popular fast-food joints.

You get extra brownie points if you actually plan your travels around food. This is completely not necessary to eating well while traveling, but it can be fun and exciting to specifically travel to a city that's known for its plant-based fare. Whether it's Vancouver, BC (where you can get a vegan hot dog at any street corner hot-dog stand); Detroit, MI (location of the world's first vegan Coney Island); or Spokane, WA (where the vegan pizza joint Allie's will ruin all of your future pizza experiences for good because nothing else will hold a candle to this), you can research where the locals eat. Look at vegan travel blogs (vegantravel.com is a perfect place to start) or search for hashtags, including #vegantravel and #veganfood, centralized to a specific area.

There are also entirely vegan travel agencies and organized vacations that specifically cater to those who want their trips to be fulfilling and delicious while avoiding meaty places; some of them even help you ensure your bedding at the hotel is free of down or feathers. Check out Vegan Epicure Travel (veganepicuretravel.com), which will set you up with destinations around the globe; VegVoyages, which offers dozens of trips throughout Asia; and definitely join VegNews Vacations (that's us!) for an all-inclusive getaway to destinations that include Paris, Thailand, India, and Mexico (vegnews.com/vacations). Another cool thing to do while traveling as a vegan is to hop around from veg B&B to B&B (both veggie-hotels. com and vegvisits.com will be your friends in this wanderlust-infused search).

If you are a self-proclaimed type A planner or if you'll be traveling through rural areas, there are two things you can do to ensure you don't go hungry: plan ahead and pack snacks. Use Google Maps, Yelp, and even Instagram (#vegancityyoutravelingin) to locate veg-friendly options before you take off. If you know you'll be hiking through the Appalachians or road-tripping across Nebraska (incidentally, home to amazing vegan restaurant Modern Love Omaha), pack snacks such as trail mix, hummus cups, and good ole PB&J.

If you're traveling with someone who is persnickety or impatient, then get a new travel buddy. Just kidding, kind of. No, but really, if you find that you're saddled with travel companions who find your veganism exhausting instead of intriguing, see whether you can create some ground rules together, including deciding to only eat at places that have options for you, or agreeing to separate for at least one meal a day so that you can try an amazing lunch or dinner at a fabulous restaurant, while your travel buddy is eating the same-old boring meat dish that will likely give them a sour stomach—but we digress. Don't let anyone dim the light of your veganism, least of all your travel companions. One of the very best parts of eating vegan is creating a sort of photo essay of your meals, so load up some apps, get your Instagram ready, and go already.

Food Flight

For the vegan jetsetter in search of plant-based food, the sky's the limit. With today's vegan options at airports nationwide, get ready to kiss your terminal hunger good-bye. Here are just a few of our favorite airport eats.

ATLANTA (ATL)
Known as the busiest airport in the United States, you may find yourself on a layover here if Atlanta isn't your final destination. Thankfully, no matter what terminal you're in, vegan options abound. From veggie burritos at Qdoba to animal-free dishes at a number of restaurants (Lotta Frutta's Viva La Vegan! Panini, The Original El Taco's Vegan Mercado Tacos, Nature's Table Vegetarian Chili, and more), you won't starve here—no matter how long your layover.

LOS ANGELES (LAX)
The City of Angels is known for its wealth of vegan options, and its airport is no exception. During your layover, devour a build-your-own wood-fired Neapolitan pizza with Daiya cheese (at no extra charge) at 800 Degrees Pizzeria, or grab a kale salad or smoothie bowl from healthy hotspot Earthbar.

NEW YORK CITY (JFK)
Korean-inspired dishes such as miso udon, tofu stew, and vegetable *bibimbap* (order without the egg) at JikJi Café have us ready to book a ticket to the Big Apple, if only for the airport experience. More of a Whole Foods hot bar fan? Cibo Express Gourmet Market comes close, complete with a salad bar, vegan-friendly hot bar, and vegan-friendly soups—all clearly labeled.

SAN FRANCISCO (SFO)
The SFO location of the popular Northern California eatery Plant Café offers everything from green curry bowls and beet burgers to trendy juices and thick smoothies to keep you full and nourished until you reach your final destination. Craving an acai or pitaya bowl topped with fresh fruit and granola? Sidewalk Juice is the place to go! And Amy's Drive Thru has everything from breakfast sandwiches to burgers and fries.

SEATTLE (SEA)
Calm pre-flight jitters with a cucumber jalapeño-infused Bloody Mary or oakey chardonnay at vegetarian restaurant Floret by Cafe Flora. Sober up with a hearty tofu scramble made with locally foraged mushrooms, delicata squash, and roasted potatoes or fried avocado with cayenne aioli.

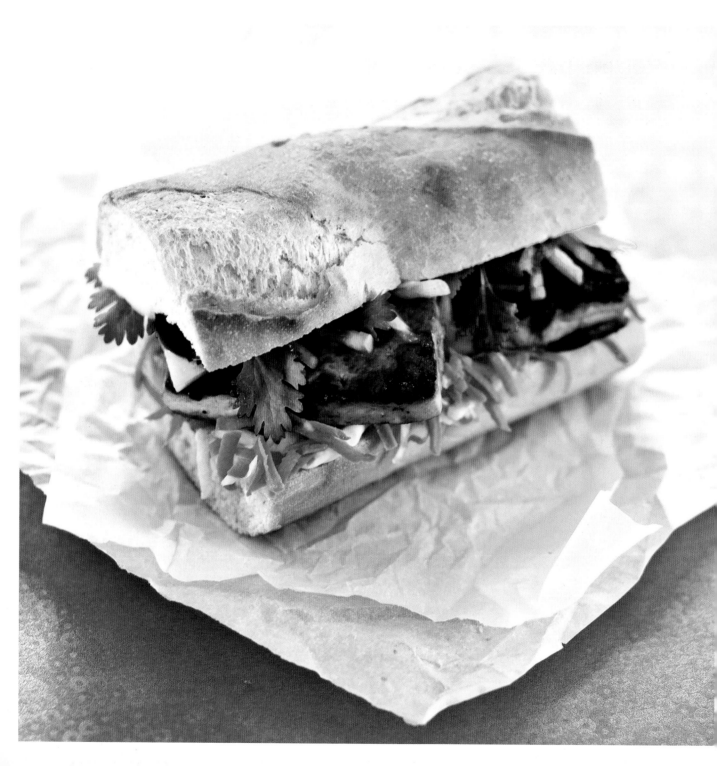

Vegan Tofu Bánh Mì

Many major cities across the country now have a local spot for vegan or veganizeable bánh mì. Now, you can make your own!

Pickles:

3   tablespoons sugar
¼   teaspoon salt
⅓   cup rice vinegar
2   tablespoons water
1   cup shredded carrot
½   cup shredded daikon

Tofu bánh mì:

2   teaspoons vegetable oil
1   pound extra-firm tofu, drained, pressed, and cut into ½-inch-thick slices

3   tablespoons hoisin sauce
2   tablespoons soy sauce
1   tablespoon sriracha sauce, plus more for serving
4   (7-inch-long) vegan baguette-style rolls
2   tablespoons vegan mayonnaise
½   English cucumber, peeled and julienned
2   tablespoons pickled jalapeño slices
1½   cups fresh cilantro leaves

❶ **Prepare the pickles:** In a bowl, whisk together sugar, salt, vinegar, and water. Add carrot and daikon and toss to coat. Cover and refrigerate for at least 1 hour. Drain completely before using.

❷ **Prepare the bánh mì:** In a skillet over medium heat, heat oil. Add tofu and cook until golden brown, turning as needed. In a small bowl, whisk together hoisin, soy sauce, and 1 teaspoon sriracha. Brush hoisin mixture over tofu, coating all sides. Remove from heat and set aside to cool.

❸ Slice baguettes lengthwise, leaving one side attached. Spread mayonnaise on both inner halves of bread, then drizzle with sriracha to taste. Layer baguettes with cucumber, tofu, pickles, jalapeño slices, and cilantro leaves. Press down top of baguettes gently and serve.

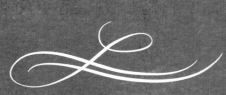

You Can Raise Vegan Kids and Not Be a Terrible Parent!

Day 28

*For many kids, animals are their friends, and respecting that important value shows that you're a terrific parent—**plus, raising a vegan child is the healthiest choice**, and way easier than you think.*

Just Google

"vegan parenting" or "raising your kids vegan" and you'll find enough resources, articles, and online forums to keep you reading until your kids are in college (but then, of course, you'd miss the opportunity to raise them, and you'd likely get reported for neglect, and the news headlines would surely point to your veganism as to why you're a neglectful parent, so don't do that). You'll find mainstream article after mainstream article that starts off skeptical ("Adults can play with their diet, but is it safe when you're dealing with children?"), but then usually pivots to the fact that raising your kids vegan is not only safe, but—assuming you're paying attention to the kids' nutritional needs (which one should do with their kids regardless of what kind of diet they're on)—it can actually be the safest and best diet, lowering their risk for allergic reactions, among other health benefits.

According to Virginia Messina, MPH, RD, and Jack Norris, RD—from their flagship book, *Vegan for Life: Everything You Need to Know to Be Healthy on a Plant-Based Diet*— "When it comes to feeding vegan children, parents need to give extra attention to vitamin B_{12}, calcium, vitamin D, and essential fats." They go on to say that similarly to grown-ups, vegan children require a reliable source of iodine and a variety of foods rich in iron, zinc, and protein. And it's as easy as that.

If you are a parent or parent-to-be, you might be rolling your eyes at the oversimplification of that statement. The truth is, it *should be* as easy as that. But there are a lot of judgmental people out there, and many societal norms that parents, in particular, will be rubbing up against. The social challenges of raising a vegan kid—or, more precisely, helping your kid navigate through living in a meat-eating world—can be more challenging than actually finding or creating food options for them.

Here are some common misperceptions, followed by the real story:

"Raising kids vegan is so much work!"

Raising kids, full stop, is so much work.

"Raising a vegan kid is so hard; I could never do it."

That's a totally normal go-to reaction, but you don't need it. Sometimes, big life decisions should be treated as a one-day-at-a-time thing. You don't need to worry about how you'll handle the holiday dinner if it's only March; you just need to figure out tonight's supper. Be easy on yourself, and trust that you'll find the answers (and the communities who will support you) as you navigate your way through your own veganism, and your kid's.

"Raising kids vegan means I'd have to cook all the time. I don't have the time."

Going vegan doesn't mean you will have a personality transplant, nor that your morning routines will change very much from what they are now. You don't have to cook any more or less than you already do (see Chapter 24). There are easy breakfasts for kids (such as plant milk and cereal, peanut butter banana toast, overnight oats, fruit smoothies, and even frozen waffles; see Chapter 4), quick grab-and-go breakfasts for busy parents (try eating what was just listed for your kids), and simple lunches you can pack that won't take much time (check out Chapter 6 for lots of ideas, but a few easy ones are packaged or homemade soups in a thermos, colorful crudités with a bean-based spread and fruit, and of course let's not forget the classic PB&J (no judgment if that happens to come in the form of the Uncrustable—yes, all but the honey varieties are vegan).

"If he's vegan, my kid won't be able to enjoy Amira's birthday party or Juan's sleepover."

The best thing to do here is to make sure you send your kid to the party with the vegan equivalent of whatever is being served. This does mean you'll need to check with the kid's parents to see what's on the menu, but due to the prevalence of allergies in children, this information is more often than not made available. You can practically bet on the food being some kind of combination of pizza, hot dogs, burgers, and cake—all of which is very easy to veganize (and if you don't have time to cook, it's not hard to find quick versions of these at most stores, which can be heated up at the party—some of our favorite vegan pizzas are made by Daiya, Sweet Earth Foods, Amy's Kitchen, and The Pizza Plant). For the cake, it might be easier to pick up for your kid a rich, vegan buttercream-dolloped cupcake (try the vegan options from Rubicon Bakers, which you can get at select Target stores, plus Whole Foods Market, Sprouts, and Safeway). But if you have time and interest, your "weirdo" kid might feel extra special if each time they go to a friend's birthday party, they have their own full cake at home—with an extra-big slice to-go for them to eat at the party itself.

"Being vegan means forcing your ideas on your kids. That's not right."

This is an interesting one, especially since that's just inherent to what it is to be a parent. If it's not right to "force your ideas on your kids," then why have kids eat meat at all? In other words, why is it the status quo to eat animals—an ethically compromised decision that also ties back to many of the diseases plaguing Western civilization—as opposed to raising kids vegan and then having them make the choice to opt into eating animals later on, should they choose, once they are aware of what it actually means to kill and eat an animal?

"My kids are such picky eaters— and they hate veggies. If they went vegan, they'd starve."

This is a tough one, for sure. One thing to keep in mind is that veganism is not about deprivation, so even though you might have the knee-jerk reaction of thinking about veganism as limiting your kids' options, we can guarantee that with a little practice

and understanding of the vegan food scene, you will soon come to see that it will do the opposite—and actually expand the food options your kid has. Transition foods (such as vegan macaroni and cheese, vegan chicken fingers, and vegan hot dogs) will be key here. And the regular "kid foods" that they're used to eating (grilled cheese, pizza, and spaghetti and meatballs) will be very easy to veganize. You will also eventually find ways of sneaking greens into your kids' meals (such as macaroni and broccoli "trees," blending veggies into pasta sauce, and sweet, fruity smoothies with a handful of spinach), which will basically award you parent of the year.

"Being a kid is hard enough. Making them vegan will make them outcast weirdos."

Like everything else, community is superimportant. So, if your kid goes to a school with no other vegans, it's a good idea to connect them with a community of other vegan kids—either through play dates on the weekends, a special vegan camp (YEA Camp is an amazing, advocacy-related summertime experience for kids aged twelve and older, and is all vegan), or by taking them to conferences and veg fests where they can meet other kids like them. It's also a fun idea to show them online videos of vegan kids (be sure to follow Genesis Butler and Greta Thunberg on Instagram, and Lean Green Dad on YouTube—and definitely follow #vegankids) so that they can start to see that they're not at all alone. As for food, if you're packing their lunches, every now and then, be sure to add something the other kids will be jealous of (such as a Justin's Dark Chocolate Peanut Butter Cup, Rule Breakers Birthday Cake Blondie, or Better Bites Bakery Cake Bite), and make the rest of their lunch box food resemble what their peers are eating (a Tofurky and vegan cheese sandwich will look no different from their classmates' sandwiches).

"Vegan kids don't get enough protein and will have stunted growth."

The protein question is not just for adults! A newly vegan kid will get their protein exactly where they used to get their protein—*from food!*—as well as where vegan adults get their protein (see Chapter 2 for a reminder). All whole foods have protein, even the plant-based variety. In fact, if your kid ate nothing but 2,000 calories of broccoli all day, they'd get a whopping 146 grams of protein. Even pasta has protein. Plain white spaghetti pasta noodles from Barilla contain 7 grams of protein per serving, and Prego's basic marinara sauce contains 2 grams of protein. And forget those three glasses of milk a day; they don't need 'em. If your kid is used to the ritual of drinking milk, swap out cows' milk for soy milk—both contain 8 grams of protein per cup, but the soy milk won't give them skin issues later down the road.

"And they won't get enough calcium, so their bones will break."

Although the dairy industry would hate to admit it, calcium is indeed available in other places besides cows' milk. Calcium-rich plant sources include beans, almonds, tofu, whole wheat bread, and enriched products, such as orange juice and cereals. But healthy bones are about more than just calcium; a plethora of nutrients are required to make strong, dense bones—such as potassium, protein, vitamin D, and magnesium. Fortunately, vegan diets that include nutrient-dense plant foods are great sources of calcium and help maintain strong bones. It's crucially important for young kids to maximize bone density, as it peaks in their teenage years. Some say that it's like a bank, and you can only make deposits in the first twenty years—but you make withdrawals for the rest of your life! So, when it comes to strong, vegan kids—all kids, really—be sure to focus on all of these nutrients.

"A vegan kid is an iron-deficient kid."

If this sounds like it's getting redundant, you're not off-track. Kids can get their iron through plants, too. Dark leafy greens, such as spinach, collard greens, and Swiss chard, are packed with iron, as are beets, lentils, beans, nuts, quinoa, figs . . . you get the idea. One tip: studies have shown that iron is better absorbed when consumed with vitamin C, so give your kid a clementine to accompany a lentil soup lunch or throw in some chopped bell pepper in a tofu and spinach scramble—dusted with plenty of cheesy nooch, of course.

Your veganism is awesome, so why not give your kid the gift of veganism too? With the exponential rise of vegans, more and more vegan babies are being born. These children develop normally, both physically and emotionally, and because they literally run on plants, they have the added benefit of running on compassion and empathy, too. Obviously, not every vegan kid (nor parent) is the same; but one commonality among so many of this new generation of people who eschew all animal products is that they are living, breathing examples of health, vitality, and a strong sense of identity and purpose.

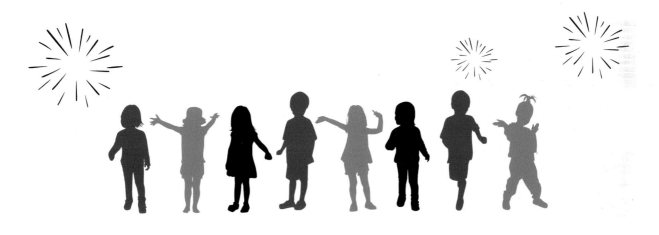

5 Ways to Make Your Kids' Vegan Bagged Lunches Ridiculously Fun

Your kid won't be made fun of for being vegan if you send them to school with amazing lunches built around these basics.

1 ADD BRIGHT COLORS

Those who can remember the '90s will recall the bizarre color trend in kid food—remember purple ketchup? Thankfully, that concoction has been discontinued, but the trend lives on. Make veggie sushi pop with carrots, avocado, and a slice of mango, and pack a sweet surprise in the form of a blue spirulina–hued vanilla pudding.

2 MAKE FUN SHAPES WITH COOKIE CUTTERS

You're going to cut the crust off anyway, so you might as well do it with a butterfly cookie cutter.

3 INCLUDE A RAINBOW OF POSSIBILITIES

Rainbows, unicorns, and mermaids—if you incorporate one of these hot topics into your kid's lunch, they'll instantly rise to lunch room royalty.

An easy way to pack a rainbow into a lunchbox is to include fruit skewers. Spear an assortment of blueberries, grapes, strawberries, kiwi slices, and pineapple or mango chunks on a wooden skewer, and bam! You've got yourself an edible rainbow.

4 SAME FOOD, DIFFERENT PRESENTATION

You don't have to reinvent the wheel or get out your crafting supplies to make your kid's bagged lunch pop. Take your standard PB&J sandwich, roll it, cut into bite-size pieces, and call it PB&J sushi. Or transform a hummus and veggie sandwich by stuffing the ingredients into a pita pocket instead.

5 HAVE FUN WITH NAMES

This tactic relies on what kids do best—use their imagination. Come up with fun names for the everyday foods in their lunchbox and label them with sticky notes. For example, call edamame "emeralds," seaweed salad "mermaid hair," or hummus "superhuman strength dip."

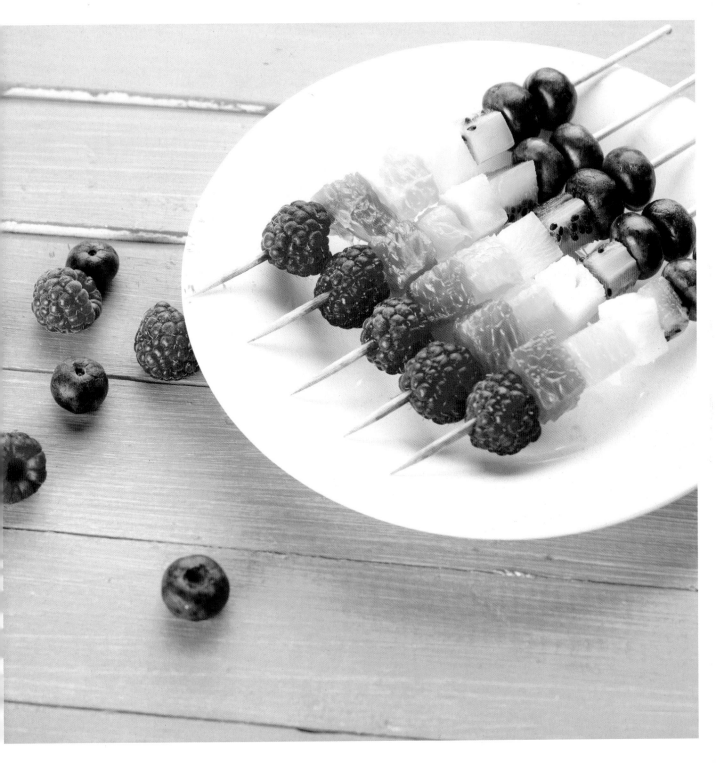

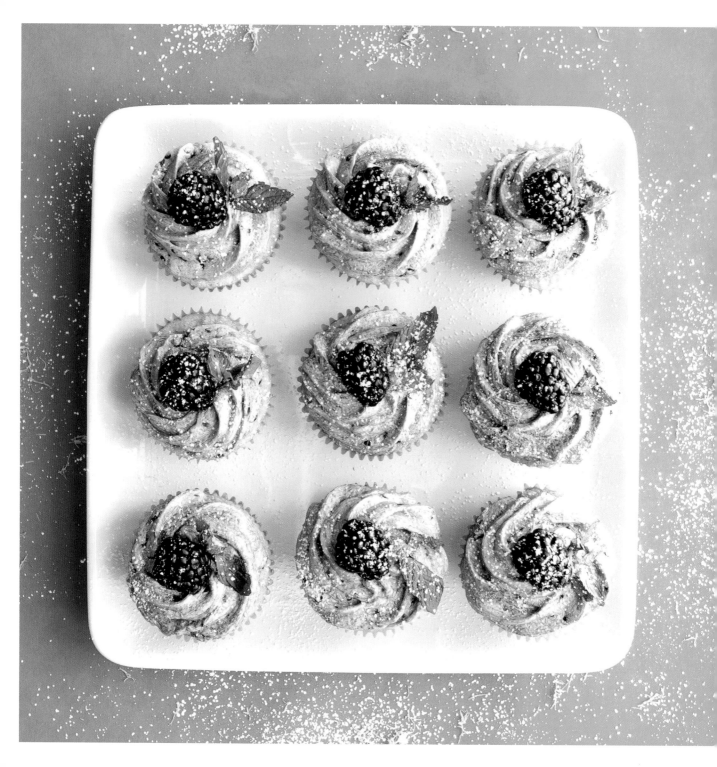

Lemon Blackberry Cupcakes

Worried your vegan kid will be an outcast? Not with these cupcakes.

Cupcakes:

1½	cups all-purpose flour
¾	cup granulated sugar
½	teaspoon baking soda
½	teaspoon baking powder
½	teaspoon salt
¾	cup water
½	cup canola oil
2	tablespoons cider vinegar
1	tablespoon lemon extract

Frosting:

1	cup vegetable shortening
2	cups powdered sugar
1	teaspoon pure vanilla extract
¼	cup fresh or frozen blackberries

Fresh blackberries, for garnish
Small mint leaves, for garnish
Powdered sugar, for dusting

❶ Prepare the cupcakes: Preheat oven to 350°F. Line two 12-well cupcake pans with 14 cupcake liners.

❷ In a large bowl, whisk together flour, granulated sugar, baking soda, baking powder, and salt. In a separate bowl, whisk together water, oil, vinegar, and lemon extract. Pour wet mixture into dry mixture and whisk until just combined, being careful not to overmix.

❸ Fill cupcake liners two-thirds full with batter. Bake for 15 to 18 minutes, or until a knife inserted in center of a cupcake comes out dry. Remove from oven and let cool completely before frosting.

❹ Prepare the frosting: Using a handheld or stand mixer, beat shortening in a large bowl until smooth. With mixer running on low speed, add powdered sugar, vanilla, and blackberries and beat to incorporate. Beat on high speed for 2 more minutes, or until light and fluffy.

❺ To assemble, frost each cupcake, garnish with blackberries and a mint leaf, and dust with powdered sugar.

No, Meat Is Not Necessary. For Literally Anyone.

Day 29

*If you have the resources to go vegan (and if you're reading this, you probably do), then one of **the best ways to fight world hunger is to go vegan**.*

The following

will happen to you at least once: you will be at that restaurant, eating that vegan option, with that friend who is eating that steak. You will be excitedly yammering on about how you're trying this new plant-based thing, and it's really working for you, and how cool is it that even this steakhouse has the Impossible burger! You'll gleefully explain how you read this book, and then you saw this documentary, and you stopped eating meat, milk, and eggs. You will tell your friend how you already feel better physically—and you feel really good that you're living in alignment with your ethics. "This is really working for me," you'll say with a smile, as you take a bite of your Impossible Burger. You'll notice that your buddy hasn't made eye contact in a hot minute, and you'll wonder if they're upset about something. You'll both *chew chew chew* for a good, long thirty seconds without saying anything, and then finally, after they swallow their last red bite of steak, they'll clear their throat, finally look you in the eye, and say, "Yeah, but what about the starving children in Africa?"

First of all, find solace in the fact that this has happened to all of us at some point, so you're in good company. Be patient with your friend as they work this through, knowing that you can vent later online in your Vegans of Oklahoma City Facebook group or what have you. Consider this conversation a rite of passage. Mazel tov!

Let's unpack this. There are definitely those who think that because they are purportedly (or optically) concerned about the "children in Africa," or any other social justice movement they deem more important than going vegan (which will be *all of them*, in that moment), that caring about animal rights (or choosing to go vegan) is somehow mutually exclusive with caring about anything else. It's true that there are a lot of pressing social and political issues to give a crap about these days, and we are definitely not placing higher importance on one versus the other. Being vegan is something you can choose to do at least three times a day as a way of voting with your dollars and boycotting cruelty. In a world where there is seemingly so little we have control over, it's gratifying to know that we have control over what we choose to consume (and not consume). And since supply is driven by demand, this makes a difference.

That doesn't mean you shouldn't care about other issues. But why not be vegan while you care about them? Oftentimes, the systems of oppression are rooted in the same place, whether you're talking about the animals or any other oppressed group. As for "starving children in Africa" specifically (and lest we forget about the starving children everywhere, including in our neighborhoods): let's just agree right now that we're not going to decide what's good for people in Africa (unless you are reading this and are in Africa); we're going to decide what's good for people in our situation, whatever that may be. And for the vast majority of us, being radically honest about the shape of the world and the resources available to us is going to point to a shift toward a plant-based diet. End of story.

Here's proof. Researchers at Lancaster University have recently deduced that the amount of crops we currently grow is sufficient to feed the burgeoning growing population—but only if we stop consuming animals. The study states that "even without improvements in crop yield, current crop production is sufficient to provide enough healthy food for the predicted 9.7 billion world population in 2050," and goes on to say, "Overall, industrialized meat and dairy production, which currently relies on feeding 34 percent of human-edible crop calories to animals globally, is highly inefficient in terms of the provision of human nutrition." The analysis found zero nutritional case for feeding human-edible crops to animals. Take a moment to take that in. Professor Nick Hewitt of the Lancaster Environment Centre said, "If society continues on a 'business-as-usual' dietary trajectory, a 119 percent increase in edible crops will be required by 2050."

These kind of gobsmacking findings are not aberrations. Research from *Proceedings of the National Academy of Sciences* found that we could feed all 327 million Americans—*plus 390 million more people!*—if we went vegan. If the land being used to produce animal products was instead used for a "nutritionally equivalent combination" of potatoes, soybeans, peanuts, and other plants, food availability would increase by 120 percent.

Of course, the issue of world hunger is complex and wouldn't be solved simply by switching the land used to grow animals to grow plants instead. According to hunger relief organization A Well-Fed World (AWFW), global hunger and food insecurity are frequently oversimplified as being primarily a problem of scarcity (not enough food) or a problem of distribution (not enough access to food). "More accurately," AWFW states, "Hunger and food insecurity result from a web of immensely complex and inter-affecting factors, including both food supply and distribution issues." Although advocates and change makers oftentimes focus on an issue narrow in its scope, AWFW believes that "while a shift toward plant-based foods is not in itself a solution to global hunger, there are immense and myriad benefits, which make it a necessary and critical component of meaningful solutions." Prioritizing plant-based agriculture

Hunger by the Numbers

41 million: The number of Americans who risk going hungry every year

821 million: The number of people worldwide who suffer from malnutrition (that's one in nine)

120 percent: The increase in total food availability if the land used for animal products were instead used for the nutritional equivalent of plant-based products

75 percent: The percentage of all agricultural land used for animal production

13 pounds: The average amount of grains required to produce a single pound of meat

for human consumption—and reducing or eliminating animal-based foods—needs to be part of that solution.

An astounding 821 million people worldwide suffer from chronic hunger, according to conservative estimates. Children suffer the most, and almost fifteen thousand of them die each day from hunger and hunger-related causes. This is nothing new. AWFW is a breath of fresh air in the realm of addressing world hunger, as it encourages the promotion of plant-based foods as necessary components of global hunger reduction and food security, working on various initiatives so that these measures can be implemented quickly and broadly.

This approach is corroborated by another study—this one from the University of Minnesota's Institute on the Environment—stating that 36 percent of the calories in crops are being fed to farmed animals. But when cattle are killed and turned into food, only 12 percent of those calories make their way into the human diet; that's a two-thirds drop in the number of calories that humans would be able to directly consume if we had eaten the grains ourselves and left the poor animals alone.

If you want to help the planet and align your day-to-day actions with your ethics, going vegan is the way to go. The UN has been reporting on the harm of animal consumption for years, as its 2006 report, "Livestock's Long Shadow," states unequivocally that the livestock sector is one of the most significant contributors to the most serious environmental problems at every scale from local to global.

So, the next time you find yourself talking with somebody who is dismissive of your veganism because they deem other issues more important—suddenly positioning themselves as world hunger advocates or experts—you might respond by validating their concern about world hunger, explaining that part of the reason you're vegan is because you're concerned about it, too, and asking them what, specifically, they're doing to address the issue. Actually, that's kind of a pretentious move. So, don't let them answer (they won't have an answer anyway, so you'd be doing them a favor). Instead, interrupt the awkward silence and see whether they want a bite of the Impossible. Then, get the check.

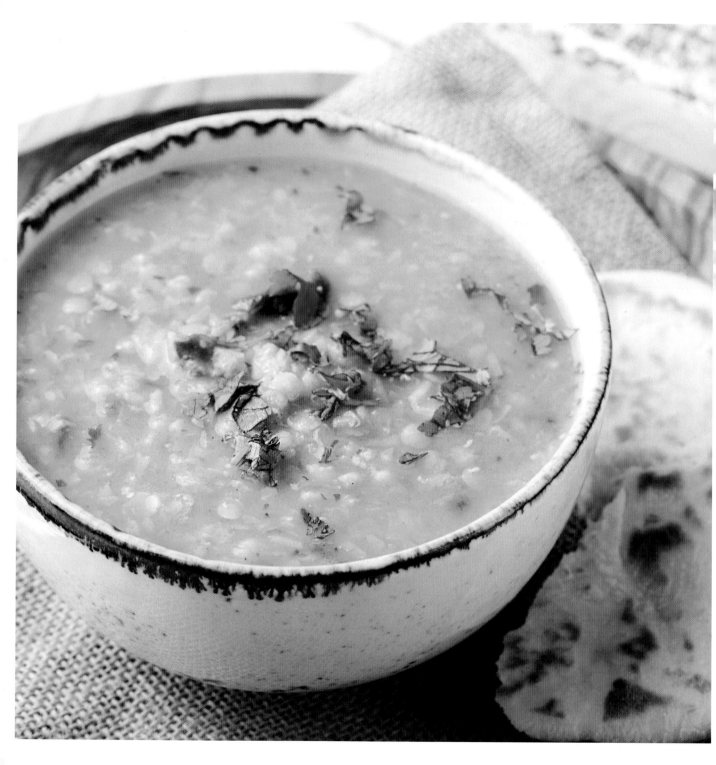

Curried Yellow Lentil Soup

Curry is among the most popular flavors in the world, while lentils are a readily available powerhouse legume filled with nutrition. Put them together, and you have a meal with universal appeal.

1	tablespoon olive oil
1	medium-size yellow onion, chopped
1	carrot, chopped
1	celery stalk, chopped
3	garlic cloves, chopped
1	cup dried yellow lentils
1	(14.5-ounce) can diced tomatoes, undrained

1½	tablespoons curry powder
1	teaspoon ground cumin
1	teaspoon ground turmeric
1	teaspoon salt
¼	teaspoon freshly ground black pepper
5	cups vegetable stock
4	cups baby spinach

❶ In a large pot over medium heat, heat olive oil. Add onion, carrot, celery, and garlic. Cover and cook for 5 minutes, or until softened. Add lentils, tomatoes, curry powder, cumin, turmeric, salt, pepper, and stock.

❷ Bring to a boil, then lower heat to a simmer. Cover and cook for 45 minutes, or until the lentils are tender, adding more stock if needed. Taste and adjust seasonings. About 5 minutes before serving, stir in spinach. Serve hot.

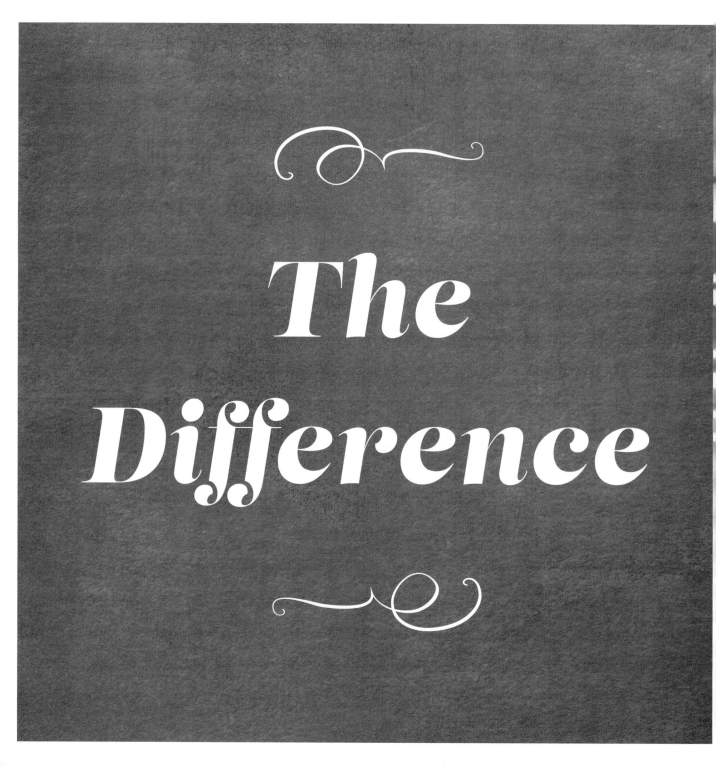

Day 30

*Social change happens person to person and by example. So, yes, if one person goes vegan, **it will and it does make a difference**.*

It can be easy

to go down the path of thinking that one person going vegan doesn't matter in the grand scheme of things. After all, this is a big world, and one person alone generally does not wield that much power

But if we thought that way about everything, we would probably not care about littering. What's the difference if one gum wrapper is on the ground? We would certainly not vote—because who cares if one person votes? It's not like it's going to change the election. If it didn't matter what one person did, then if we had the means, we might get an additional car—not worrying about whether it's gas-guzzling. We'd buy the Styrofoam cups—not the recyclable ones—for kids' birthday parties. Actually, why recycle at all? After all, we're just one person; we're not going to make or break any systems all by ourselves. Bring on the steak!

But there's a lot more to it than that, and social change still happens person to person and by example. So if you're at the grocery store and you ask where the Beyond Meat burgers are, you're not only just affecting that store by buying the Beyond Meat and showing that there's a demand for that product, but you're also opening the eyes of the person whom you're asking. Someone else nearby you hears "Beyond Meat" and they think, *"huh . . . "* Next time they are in the section of the grocery store with those burgers, they might just pick them up.

Similarly, if you're at a restaurant and you order the vegan meal, the server, chef, and manager are all hearing you in one way or another, and they know there's an interest in vegan food. Plus, the person at the table next to you—or maybe your nonvegan dining-mate sitting across from you—hears, sees, and (if you're the sharing type) perhaps tastes that as well.

We are influencing people *constantly*, all the time, in ways that we can't possibly understand. So, just by living our lives and being true to our values, our efforts go far, far beyond us. Plus, by buying the Beyond Meat patties or ordering that vegan item at the restaurant, we are also affecting the bottom line—and, of course, supply is driven by demand—so your choices make way, way more of a difference than it might seem.

There's also this: every life matters. It's like that poignant, albeit overused starfish story (originally adapted from "The Star Thrower" essay by Loren Eiseley), which you probably already know (it's overused for a reason), but the short version goes something like this: boy goes to beach and sees a lot of starfish washed up by the waves; boy starts to pick them up one by one and tosses them back into the ocean; man comes by and points out that there are too many starfish for him to save and it won't make a difference, saying, "You can't save them all, so why bother trying?"; boy thinks about this and responds, "Well, it matters to this one," and then flings the starfish back into the giant sea.

Every individual life matters. No matter who you are and how much you say that what you do doesn't matter, the fact it is, *it does*; everyone's individual actions matter a lot. They not only directly matter (such as to that one starfish—or cow, pig, or chicken), but since we are a highly impressionable, social species, our actions have the power to normalize or inspire others.

Let's assume you're down with all of that—that you recognize that our choices make a difference.

It's also important to remember that you don't have to fix everything to fix *something*. If you save just one animal from suffering, it's worth it; that alone is worth every moment of your effort.

Serious crises are looming (and upon us already) that are going to enormously change the way we consume food. Climate change, land use, pollution—all of these are contributing to our understanding that things have got to change. If we listen to the folks worth listening to, we will find that the way we eat now just isn't sustainable. Not eating meat is a twofold win: (1) it can slow the destructive path we're on, and (2) it will help make vegan food more accessible. Every single person who purchases plant-based instead of animal-based is therefore making an enormous change. Supporting these foods is a strong, political act—and so is boycotting foods that are cruel, unsustainable, and unhealthy.

Yes, we need systemic solutions; but the best way to motivate business and government is to vote with our dollars. Even in small towns and cities across the United States and the globe, more and more vegan places are popping up—from Kansas City to Spokane to Colorado Springs, and everywhere in between. There are also more and more vegan companies, animal-rights advocates, food scientists, and financial investors working to ensure that our collective future is both compassionate and delicious.

There is no way these businesses would be making the changes they are making—major fast-food chains introducing vegan options, vegan meat companies going public and the stocks skyrocketing, plant-based milk innovations growing exponentially—if one person had not initially gone vegan. And then another. And then another. It really is pretty simple, when you get down to it.

The important thing is to not let other people get in your way, and there will always be the naysayers. But you've made it this far, so you probably already know that if you listen to naysayers your whole life, you'll never do anything you want to do— or anything that matters. Beyond them, though, try as best you can to not be your own naysayer, and not get in your own damn way. The arguments you make with yourself about veganism are solvable, and are ultimately not that important when compared with the deep satisfaction you can get from really making this change and sticking the dismount.

Once you do, you'll find that it's 100 percent positive. You'll meet wonderful people, taste incredible food, be connected with a deeper purpose, and have a whole lot of fun. Most important, you'll be out there shining in your corner of this world, knowing deep down that you're doing your absolute best, and living your own, beautiful truth in your one, glorious life. Enjoy the ride.

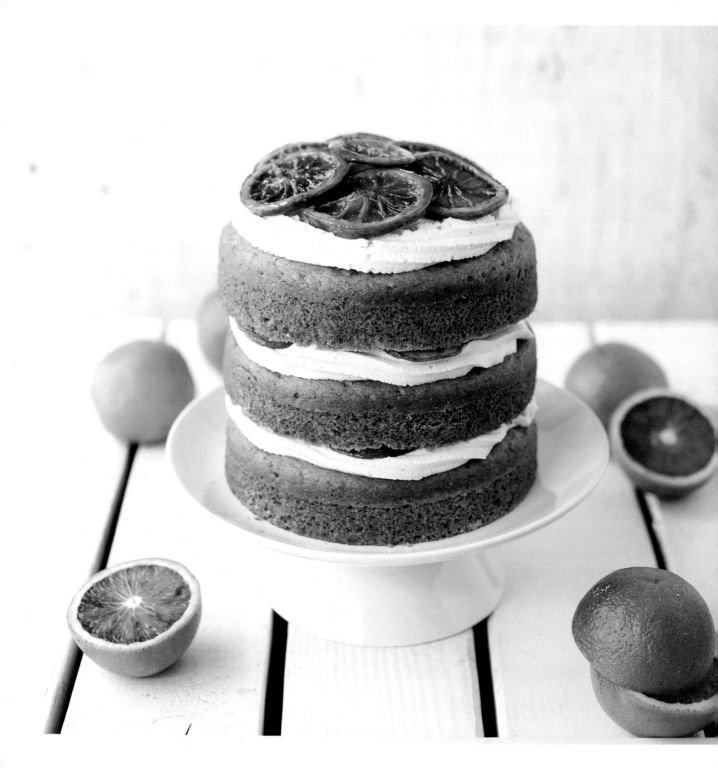

Candied Blood Orange Cake with Vanilla Bean Buttercream

Serves 8

Celebrate the good life with this showstopping dessert featuring fragrant, orange-infused cake, fluffy vanilla bean–flecked frosting, and candied blood orange slices.

Cake:
Cooking spray, for pans
1½ cups all-purpose flour
1   cup whole wheat pastry flour
2   teaspoons baking soda
½   teaspoon salt
1   cup ice-cold water
1   cup granulated sugar
½   cup applesauce
½   cup freshly squeezed blood orange juice
¼   cup olive oil
2   tablespoons white vinegar
1   teaspoon orange zest
1   teaspoon orange extract

Frosting:
¾   cup vegan butter
2½   cups powdered sugar
1   vanilla bean, seeds scraped and reserved
1   teaspoon pure vanilla extract

Candied blood orange slices:
2   blood oranges, unpeeled, sliced into 14 rounds
¼   cup granulated sugar

❶ **Prepare the cake:** Preheat oven to 325°F. Spray three 6-inch round cake pans lightly with cooking spray. In a large bowl, sift together flours, baking soda, and salt. In a medium-size bowl, whisk together remaining cake ingredients.

❷ Pour wet mixture into dry mixture and whisk until smooth. Divide batter equally among prepared cake pans. Bake for 25 to 30 minutes, or until a knife inserted into center of cake comes out clean. Remove from oven and let cool on a wire rack for at least 1 hour before removing from pans, then set aside.

❸ **Prepare the frosting:** Using a hand mixer on high speed, whip butter in a bowl. Continue to whip while adding powdered sugar, ½ cup at a time, until all is incorporated. Add vanilla bean seeds and vanilla extract and whip until evenly combined. Place frosting in refrigerator until ready to assemble.

❹ **Prepare the candied blood orange slices:** In a large skillet over medium heat, arrange blood orange slices in a single layer and sprinkle with sugar. Bring to a simmer and adjust heat to medium-low, flipping after 5 minutes. Cook until slices have softened and all excess liquid has evaporated. Transfer slices to a parchment paper–lined plate to cool.

5 To assemble the cake, use a hand mixer at high speed to whip frosting for 5 minutes. Place one cake layer on a serving plate or cake stand. Using a piping bag or offset spatula, place a ½-inch layer of frosting onto top of first cake layer. Arrange four candied blood orange slices on top of frosting, then top with second layer of cake.

6 Repeat, finally, topping with third layer of cake. Pipe remaining frosting on top of cake, and arrange remaining candied blood orange slices on frosting in a circular, overlapping fashion. Serve immediately or refrigerate until ready to serve.

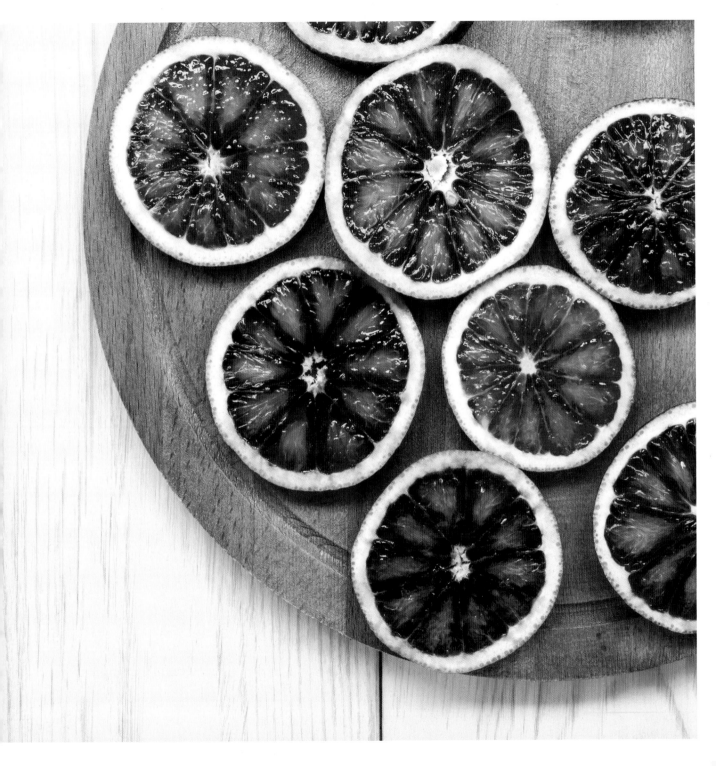

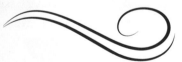

References

CHAPTER 1

3 *I had been a participant:* Dick Gregory and Sheila P. Moses, *Callus on My Soul: A Memoir* (New York: Dafina, 2003).

CHAPTER 2

7 *plant protein can meet:* "Position of the American Dietetic Association and the Dietitians of Canada: Vegetarian Diets," *Journal of the American Dietetic Association* 103, no. 6 (June 2003): 748–765.

7 *way too much protein:* Micah Dorfner, "Are You Getting Too Much Protein?" Mayo Clinic News Network, February 23, 2017, https://newsnetwork.mayoclinic.org/discussion/are-you-getting-too-much-protein/.

7 *Kwashiorkor:* Natalie Butler and the Healthline Editorial Team, "What Is Kwashiorkor?" 2017, https://www.healthline.com/health/kwashiorkor.

7 *Vegans specifically get protein:* Alice Petre, "The 17 Best Protein Sources for Vegans and Vegetarians," 2016, https://www.healthline.com/nutrition/protein-for-vegans-vegetarians.

8 *twenty different amino acids:* "Protein Structure," Scitable, Nature Education, n.d., https://www.nature.com/scitable/topicpage/protein-structure-14122136.

8 *antiquated idea:* Physicians Committee for Responsible Medicine, "Dr. Neal Barnard: Can Vegans Get Enough Protein?" uploaded September 12, 2017, YouTube, https://www.youtube.com/watch?v=ukY5_VFcA08.

8 *Adults should eat 0.36 grams:* Daniel Pendick, "How Much Protein Do You Need Every Day?" *Harvard Health Blog* (blog). June 25, 2019, https://www.health.harvard.edu/blog/how-much-protein-do-you-need-every-day-201506188096.

8 *The meat industrial complex:* Michele Simon, "Protein Propaganda: It's What's for Dinner," Grist, February 1, 2012, https://grist.org/food/protein-propaganda-its-whats-for-dinner.

CHAPTER 3

13 *Diets come and go:* Vegan Society, "History," 2019, https://www.vegansociety.com/about-us/history.

13 *Plant-based companies in Brazil:* Sociedade Vegetariana Brasileira, "IBOPE Survey Shows Historical Growth in the Number of Vegetarians in the Country," 2018, https://www.svb.org.br/2473-vegetarians-in-brazil.

13 *In China, the vegan population:* TimeOut Beijing, "Life on the Veg: Rise of Vegetarianism in China," 2017, http://www.timeoutbeijing.com/features

/Living_in_Beijing/162166/Life-on-the-veg-the
-rise-of-vegetarianism-in-China-.html.

13 *Germany is leading the way:* Meera Senthilingam, "Are Germans Leading a Vegan Revolution?" CNN, July 31, 2017, https://www.cnn.com/2017/05/03/health/germany-vegan-vegetarian-diets/index.html.

14 *In Canada:* Mintel Press Team, "More Than Half of Canadians Eat Meat Alternatives," 2008, https://www.mintel.com/press-centre/food-and-drink/positive-future-for-plant-proteins-more-than-half-of-canadians-eat-meat-alternatives.

14 *In the United Kingdom:* Rachel Moss, "3.5 Million People in the UK Are Now Vegan," Huffington Post, April 4, 2018, https://www.huffingtonpost.co.uk.

14 *by the time Miley Cyrus:* NYU Arts & Science, Animal Studies MA Program, 2018, https://www.nyu.edu/fas/email/animalstudies/index_browser.html.

14 *Veganism has deep roots:* "African Vegans Are a Return to Tradition," *This Is Africa* (blog), August 2, 2017, https://thisisafrica.me/politics-and-society/african-vegans-return-tradition/.

14 *whether the global shift:* Felicity Carus, "UN Urges Global Move to Meat and Dairy-Free Diet," *Guardian*, June 2, 2010, https://www.theguardian.com/environment/2010/jun/02/un-report-meat-free-diet.

CHAPTER 4

20 *In China:* Ailbhe Malone, "This Is What Breakfast Looks Like in 22 Countries Around the World,"

BuzzFeed, February 6, 2015, https://www.buzzfeed.com/ailbhemalone/breakfasts-around-the-world.

CHAPTER 5

27 *can fall short on fiber:* Diane Quagliani and Patricia Felt-Gunderson, "Closing America's Fiber Intake Gap: Communication Strategies from a Food and Fiber Summit," *American Journal of Lifestyle Medicine* 11, no. 1 (January–February 2017): 80–85, https://www.ncbi.nlm.nih.gov/pmc/articles/PMC6124841/.

27 *As for vegans:* There's the B_{12} question, and B_{12} should be supplemented. Note, though, that the reason it requires supplementation at all is that it is made from bacteria which used to be available from the soil and vegetables. But the advent of modern hygiene has taken that away, which is why it's now only available in trace amounts through an animal's intestinal tract—but it's extremely inefficient, in that consuming B_{12} that way also gives you cholesterol and bad fat, and many people's body can't absorb B_{12} that way anyhow. So, take a damn vitamin and move on (you can also get it from nutritional yeast and fortified plant-based milks). Shivam Joshi, "Why Every Vegan and Vegetarian Needs Vitamin B_{12}," *Forks Over Knives* (blog). March 19, 2019, https://www.forksoverknives.com/every-vegan-vegetarian-needs-vitamin-b12/#gs.ncrbe8.

CHAPTER 6

33 *Anglo-Saxon word* nuncheon: Sherrie McMillan, What Time Is Dinner," *History Magazine*, September

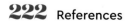

/October 2001, http://www.history-magazine.com/dinner2.html.

35 *all 1,700 public schools:* Doug Criss, "New York Public Schools to Have 'Meatless Mondays' Starting This Fall," CNN, March 12, 2019, https://www.cnn.com/2019/03/12/us/new-york-meatless-mondays-trnd/index.html.

35 *provide funding to schools*: AB-479 School meals: plant-based food and milk options, California School Plant-Based Food and Beverage Program. 2019, https://leginfo.legislature.ca.gov/faces/billHistoryClient.xhtml?bill_id=201920200AB479.

35 *Lunchables inventor:* Keith Loria, "Improved Nature Raises $3m to Launch Plant-Based Protein Company," *AgFunder News*, September 18, 2018, https://agfundernews.com/breaking-exclusive-improved-nature-raises-5m-to-launch-plant-based-protein-company.html.

CHAPTER 7

43 *more than twenty three million people:* Robyn Correll and Jason DelCollo, "Food Deserts," *Verywell Health* (blog), November 28, 2019, https://www.verywellhealth.com/what-are-food-deserts-4165971.

CHAPTER 8

49 Carbs *give you energy:* U.S. Anti-Doping Agency (USADA), "Carbohydrates—The Master Fuel," 2019, https://www.usada.org/resources/nutrition/carbohydrates-the-master-fuel/.Carbs.

50 *carbs with a bit of protein:* Jack Norris and Virginia Messina, *Vegan for Life: Everything You Need to Know to Be Healthy and Fit on a Plant-Based Diet* (Cambridge, MA: Da Capo Press, 2011).

50 *fats are a form of energy:* Sylvie Tremblay and Jill Coreone, "Fat Burning vs. Carbohydrate Burning," *Livestrong* (blog), May 30, 2019, https://www.livestrong.com/article/32587-fat-burning-vs.-carbohydrate-burning/.

50 *0.36 grams of protein:* U.S. Anti-Doping Agency (USADA), "Protein's Role as a Team Player," 2019, https://www.usada.org/resources/nutrition/proteins-role-as-a-team-player/.

50 *micronutrients and antioxidants:* Switch4Good,"Top 10 Dairy-Free Foods to Fuel Athletes," 2020, https://switch4goodsoccer.org/Top-10-Dairy-Free-Foods-to-Fuel-Athletes/.

50 *potatoes and white beans:* Sharon O'Brien, "15 Foods That Pack More Potassium Than a Banana," *Healthline*, July 26, 2019, https://www.healthline.com/nutrition/foods-loaded-with-potassium#section1.

51 *strength training comprises:* Jack Norris, "Weightlifting for Vegans," *Vegan Health: Evidence-Based Nutrient Recommendations* (blog), 2018, https://veganhealth.org/vegan-weightlifting/.

CHAPTER 10

65 *sixteen commitments:* United Nations Framework Convention on Climate Change (UNFCCC), *Fashion Industry Charter for Climate Action*, 2018, https://unfccc.int/climate-action/sectoral-engagement

/global-climate-action-in-fashion/about-the-fashion-industry-charter-for-climate-action.

66 *majority of leather:* Food and Agriculture Organization of the United Nations, "World Statistical Compendium on Raw Hides and Skins, Leather and Leather Footwear 1999–2015," 2016, http://www.fao.org/3/a-i5599e.pdf.

66 *fashion mecca:* "Prohibiting the sale of fur apparel," 2019 (New York City) Version A, https://legistar.council.nyc.gov/LegislationDetail.aspx?ID=3903503&GUID=EBE55293-8737-4620-945A-308ADC3A23DC&Options=ID|Text|&Search=1476.

67 *More than 50 percent of fur:* Clay Hales, "China's Fur Capital Touts Itself to World Even If Fur's Out at Versace and Other Leading Fashion Houses," *South China Morning Post*, March 18, 2018, https://www.scmp.com/lifestyle/fashion-beauty/article/2137458/chinas-fur-capital-touts-itself-world-even-if-furs-out.

67 *Chinese fur is often mislabeled:* Humane Society International, "T K MAXX, Boohoo, Not On The High Street Among Online Retail Giants Caught Selling Real Fur Advertised as 'Faux,'" 2017, https://www.hsi.org/news-media/online-real-as-faux-122017/.

67 *several big companies: The Humane Society of the United States vs. Andrew & Suzanne Co. Inc. DBA Andrew Marc, et al.,* 2008, "Before the United States Federal Trade Commission: Supplemental Petition to Enjoin False Advertising and Labeling of Fur Garments and to Impose Civil and Criminal Penalities," 2008, https://www.humanesociety.org/sites/default/files/docs/ftc-supplemental-petition.pdf.

67 *3D-printed fur alternatives:* Christine Flammia, "Real Fur Is Bad for Animals. Fake Fur Is Bad for the Earth. What the Hell Do We Do Now?" *Esquire*, January 17, 2019, https://www.esquire.com/style/mens-fashion/a22565653/faux-fur-real-fur/.

67 *Over a hundred million animals:* Humane Society International, "The Fur Trade," 2019, https://www.hsi.org/news-media/fur-trade/.

68 *2.25 million adult and baby sheep:* "Flystrike in Sheep," *Franklin Vets* (blog), November 15, 2017, https://franklinvets.co.nz/2017/11/15/flystrike-in-sheep/.

CHAPTER 11

76 *The bones originate from cows:* PETA, *FAQ: Are animal ingredients included in white sugar?* https://www.peta.org/about-peta/faq/are-animal-ingredients-included-in-white-sugar/.

76 *In her book,* Sweet + Salty: Lagusta Yearwood, *Sweet + Salty: The Art of Vegan Chocolates, Truffles,Caramels, and More from Lagusta's Luscious* (New York: Da Capo Lifelong Books, 2019).

CHAPTER 12

84 *more than 800,000 animals:* USDA Animal and Plant Health Inspection Service, *Annual Report Animal Usage by Fiscal Year (Fiscal Year: 2017)*, https://www.aphis.usda.gov/animal_welfare/downloads/reports/Annual-Report-Animal-Usage-by-FY2017.pdf.

84 *$12 billion:* Justin Goodman, "GenOpp: How the Government Is Perpetuating $12 Billion in Animal

Cruelty," *White Coat Waste Project* (blog), July 14, 2015, https://blog.whitecoatwaste.org/2015/07/14/genoppinterview/.

84 *Draize test:* "Dear EarthTalk: Do Cosmetic Companies Still Test on Live Animals?" *Earthtalk* 20, no. 4 (July/August 2009), https://www.scientificamerican.com/article/cosmetics-animal-testing/.

84 *RASAR:* Thomas Luechtefeld, Dan Marsh, Craig Rowlands, and Thomas Hartung, "Machine Learning of Toxicological Big Data Enables Read-Across Structure Activity Relationships (RASAR) Outperforming Animal Test Reproducibility," *Toxicological Sciences* 165, no. 1 (September 2018): 198–212, https://www.ncbi.nlm.nih.gov/pmc/articles/PMC6135638/.

CHAPTER 13

92 *cheese is not necessarily:* Rebecca Orchant, "Bad News: These 11 Cheeses Aren't Always Vegetarian," *Huffington Post*, December 19, 2013, https://www.huffpost.com/entry/vegetarian-cheese-animal-rennet_n_4467430.

92 *milk has 0.2 grams of trans fat:* American Heart Association, "Trans Fats," 2017, https://www.heart.org/en/healthy-living/healthy-eating/eat-smart/fats/trans-fat.

92 *unregulated cell growth:* Panagiotis F. Christopoulos, Pavlos Msaouel, and Michael Koutsilieris, "The Role of the Insulin-like Growth Factor-1 System in Breast Cancer," *Molecular Cancer* 14, no. 1 (February 15, 2015): 43, https://doi.org/10.1186/s12943-015-0291-7.

93 *African, Asian, Hispanic, and Indigenous:* Susan S. Lang, "Lactose Intolerance Seems Linked to Ancestral Struggles with Harsh Climate and Cattle Diseases, Cornell Study Finds," *Cornell Chronicle*, June 1, 2005, https://news.cornell.edu/stories/2005/06/lactose-intolerance-linked-ancestral-struggles-climate-diseases.

93 *you save the water equivalent:* Institution of Mechanical Engineers, "Food Waste Report—Data," 2013, https://docs.google.com/spreadsheets/d/1nzLDn1LbiwVe2TL4y4kiejuUQKpIx4Z3R5GHOguwvmo/edit#gid=0; "Gallons Used Per Person Per Day." City of Philadelphia, accessed July 7, 2019, https://www.phila.gov/water/educationoutreach/Documents/Homewateruse_IG5.pdf.

93 *legal amount of pus:* Michael Greger, "How Much Pus Is There in Milk?" NutritionFacts.org, September 8, 2011, https://nutritionfacts.org/2011/09/08/how-much-pus-is-there-in-milk/.

CHAPTER 14

99 *serious autoimmune disease affects:* Sarah Klein, "9 Things You Should Know Before Going Gluten-Free," *Huffington Post*, February 4, 2014, https://www.huffpost.com/entry/know-before-going-gluten-free_n_4719554?ir=Healthy+Living.

100 *a "nutritarian diet":* Dr. Fuhrman, "The Nutritarian Diet: Live Longer. Live Better," 2020, https://www.drfuhrman.com/.

CHAPTER 15

108 *breeding flocks:* Vegan Peace, "Down and Feathers," 2015, http://www.veganpeace.com/animal_cruelty/downandfeathers.htm.

CHAPTER 16

114 *lower breast cancer risk:* A. H. Wu, M. C. Yu, C.-C. Tseng, and M. C. Pike, "Epidemiology of Soy Exposures and Breast Cancer Risk," *British Journal of Cancer*, 98 (2008): 9–14, https://www.nature.com/articles/6604145.pdf.

115 *daily recommended amount of fiber:* Mayo Clinic Staff, "How to Add More Fiber to Your Diet," Mayo Clinic, November 16, 2018, https://www.mayoclinic.org/healthy-lifestyle/nutrition-and-healthy-eating/in-depth/fiber/art-20043983.

115 *Ninety-five percent of Americans:* Jennifer Hyland, "Fast Fiber Facts: What It Is and How to Get Enough," *U.S. News & World Report*, August 22, 2018, https://health.usnews.com/health-care/for-better/articles/2018-08-22/fast-fiber-facts-what-it-is-and-how-to-get-enough.

CHAPTER 17

121 *fifteen members:* Cameron Wolfe, "Vegan Meals All the Rage for Titans, with 15 Players Converted," *ESPN* (blog), August 8, 2018, https://www.espn.com/blog/tennessee-titans/post/_/id/26419/vegan-meals-all-the-rage-for-titans-with-15-players-converted.

CHAPTER 18

127 *one pound of beef:* Jonathan Parks-Ramage, "1,800 Gallons of Water Goes into One Pound of Meat," *Vice*, June 2 2017, https://www.vice.com/en_us/article/d3z8az/1800-gallons-of-water-goes-into-one-pound-of-meat.

128 *leading cause of deforestation:* Climate Nexus. "Animal Agriculture's Impact on Climate Change," https://climatenexus.org/climate-issues/food/animal-agricultures-impact-on-climate-change/.

128 *up to 83 percent of farmland:* Matthew Zampa, "The Problem with Farming Animals," *Sentient Media*, September 17, 2019, https://sentientmedia.org/the-problem-with-farming-animals/.

128 *two billion tons of manure:* "Animal Agriculture," *Footprints for the Future* (blog), https://footprints.earthday.org/animal-agriculture/.

128 *over a 100-year period:* David Suzuki Foundation, "Methane Pollution," 2020, https://davidsuzuki.org/project/methane-pollution/.

128 *biggest contributor of methane:* Food and Agriculture Organization of the United Nations, "GLEAM 2.0—Assessment of Greenhouse Gas Emissions and Mitigation Potential," 2020, http://www.fao.org/gleam/results/en/#c303615.

128 *replacing beef with plants:* Becca Koblin, "Veganism and Climate Change: How Eating a Plant-Based Diet Can Decrease Your Carbon Footprint," *Medium*, March 13, 2019, https://medium.com/nj-spark/veganism-and-climate-change-how-eating-a-plant-based-diet-can-decrease-your-carbon-footprint-f3e5a87d24.

CHAPTER 19

135 *most people need 66 days:* Phillippa Lally, Cornelia H. M. van Jaarsveld, Henry W. W. Potts, and Jane Wardle, "How Are Habits Formed: Modelling Habit Formation in the Real World,"

European Journal of Social Psychology 40, no. 6 (October 2010): 998–1009, https://doi.org/10.1002/ejsp.674.

CHAPTER 20

143 *seventy billion per year:* "Facts: Farm Animals," Animal Matters, 2020, http://www.animalmatters.org/facts/farm/.

143 *trillions of fish:* Michael Pellman Rowland, "Two-Thirds of the World's Seafood Is Over-Fished—Here's How You Can Help," *Forbes*, July 25, 2017, https://www.forbes.com/sites/michaelpellmanrowland/2017/07/24/seafood-sustainability-facts/.

144 *they cool off in the mud:* Henry Nicholls, "The Truth About Pigs," BBC, September 24, 2015, http://www.bbc.com/earth/story/20150924-the-truth-about-pigs.

144 *vast majority of animals killed:* United Poultry Concerns, "Poultry Slaughter: The Need for Legislation," 2019, https://www.upc-online.org/slaughter/poultry_slaughter.pdf.

145 *300 million turkeys:* Piedmont Farm Animal Refuge, "Turkeys Used for Meat," 2019, http://piedmontrefuge.org/turkeys-used-for-meat/.

145 *considered smarter than dogs:* PETA, "Pigs: Intelligent Animals Suffering on Farms and in Slaughterhouses," 2020, https://www.peta.org/issues/animals-used-for-food/animals-used-food-factsheets/pigs-intelligent-animals-suffering-factory-farms-slaughterhouses/.

146 *cows raised for meat:* PETA, "The Beef Industry," 2020, https://www.peta.org/issues/animals-used-for-food/factory-farming/cows/beef-industry/.

146 *animals are frequently exported:* Compassion in World Farming, "The Global Live Animal Transport Trade," 2020, https://www.ciwf.org.uk/our-campaigns/live-animal-transport/global-live-animal-transport-trade/.

147 *salmon can remember:* Fish Feel, "Fish Feel," 2020, http://fishfeel.org/.

147 *aquaculture output:* Let Fish Live, "Fish Who Are Farmed," http://letfishlive.org/.

147 *Nearly half of the fish:* PETA, "Aquafarming," 2020, https://www.peta.org/issues/animals-used-for-food/factory-farming/fish/aquafarming/.

CHAPTER 21

154 *Words like cage-free:* Stephanie Strom, "What to Make of Those Animal-Welfare Labels on Meat and Eggs," *New York Times*, January 31, 2017, https://www.nytimes.com/2017/01/31/dining/animal-welfare-labels.html and http://www.humanemyth.org/.

154 *Twenty-Eight Hour Law:* Twenty Eight Hour Law, U.S. Code 49 (1994), §80502, https://www.animallaw.info/statute/us-food-animal-twenty-eight-hour-law.

154 *USDA standard:* USDA Agricultural Marketing Service, "Guidelines for Organic Certification of Poultry," https://www.ams.usda.gov/sites/default/files/media/Poultry%20-%20Guidelines.pdf.

155 *many humane-sounding labels:* A Well-Fed World, "Humane Slaughter?" https://humanefacts.org/humane-slaughter/.

155 *If you're not a bird:* Farm Sanctuary, "The Truth Behind Humane Labels," https://www.farmsanctuary.org/learn/factory-farming/the-truth-behind-humane-labels/.

155 *Kosher and halal:* Bill Gardner, "Sharp Rise in Halal Abattoirs Slaughtering Animals Without Stunning Them First," *Telegraph*, January 29, 2015, https://www.telegraph.co.uk/news/religion/11378667/Sharp-rise-in-halal-abattoirs-slaughtering-animals-without-stunning-them-first.html; Animal Legal Defense Fund, "Kosher Slaughter Laws and an End to "Shackle-and-Hoist" Restraint," January 24, 2015, https://aldf.org/article/kosher-slaughter-laws-and-an-end-to-shackle-and-hoist-restraint/.

155 *sent through the mail:* "Hazardous, Restricted, and Perishable Mail: Live Animals," US Post Office Publication 52 §526.3, https://pe.usps.com/text/pub52/pub52c5_008.htm#ep184002.

CHAPTER 22

161 *on the dietary guidelines:* US Department of Agriculture, "MyPlate, MyState," https://www.choosemyplate.gov/myplate-mystate.

161 *According to the* Washington Post: Arthur Allen, "U.S. Touts Fruit and Vegetables While Subsidizing Animals That Become Meat," *Washington Post*, October 3, 2011, https://www.washingtonpost.com/national/health-science/us-touts-fruit-and-vegetables-while-subsidizing-animals-that-become-meat/2011/08/22/gIQATFG5IL_story.html?utm_term=.cf3f4c7b3c64.

162 *Meatonomics:* David Robinson Simon, "The Meatonomic$ Index," *Meatonomics* (blog), August 23, 2013, https://meatonomics.com/2013/08/22/meatonomics-index/.

CHAPTER 23

167 *First, the ugly: it's true:* Hillary Eaton, "There's Blood and Bladders in Your Wine," *Vice*, June 3, 2015, https://www.vice.com/en_us/article/ypxjzg/theres-blood-and-bladders-in-your-wine.

167 *Biodynamic wine follows a practice:* Biodynamic Association, "Who Was Rudolf Steiner?" https://www.biodynamics.com/steiner.html.

168 Can *biodynamic wine be made vegan?:* Sunny Gandara, "Italian Winery Querciabella Leading the Way in Vegan, Biodynamic an Organic Winemaking," *Sunny Gandara* (blog), September 6, 2018, https://sunnygandara.com/italian-winery-querciabella-leading-the-way-in-vegan-biodynamic-and-organic-winemaking/.

CHAPTER 26

185 *erectile disfunction affects:* National Institute of Diabetes and Digestive and Kidney Diseases," "How Common Is Erectile Dysfunction?" 2017, https://www.niddk.nih.gov/health-information/urologic-diseases/erectile-dysfunction/definition-facts#common.

185 *reduce the buildup of plaque:* Neal Barnard, "Six Reasons Athletes Are Running Toward a Vegan Diet," *Physicians Committee for Responsible Medicine* (blog), January 10, 2019, https://www

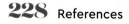

.pcrm.org/news/blog/six-reasons-athletes-are -running-toward-vegan-diet.

185 *nearly one-third of participants:* K. Esposito, F. Giugliano, C. Di Palo, G. Giugliano, R. Marfella, F. D'Andrea, M. D'Armiento, and D. Giugliano, "Effect of Lifestyle Changes on Erectile Dysfunction in Obese Men: A Randomized Controlled Trial," *JAMA* 291, no. 24 (2004): 2978–2984, https:// www.ncbi.nlm.nih.gov/pubmed/15213209.

185 *men who eat vegan meals:* Jan Havlicek and Pavlina Lenochova, "The Effect of Meat Consumption on Body Odor Attractiveness," *Chemical Senses* 31, no. 8 (October 2006): 747–752, https://www .ncbi.nlm.nih.gov/pubmed/16891352.

186 *Dr. De-Lin recommends:* Stacy De-Lin, "VegHealth." *VegNews*, issue 119 (Summer 2019): 80–81.

CHAPTER 28

197 *According to Virginia Messina:* Jack Norris and Virginia Messina, *Vegan for Life: Everything You Need to Know to Be Healthy on a Plant-Based Diet* (New York: Da Capo Lifelong Books, 2011).

CHAPTER 29

208 *crops we currently grow:* M. Berners-Lee, C. Kennelly, R. Watson, and C. N. Hewitt, "Current Global Food Production Is Sufficient to Meet Human Nutritional Needs in 2050 Provided There Is Radical Societal Adaptation," *Elementa Science of the Anthopocene* 6, no. 1 (July 2018): 52, https://www.elementascience.org/article /10.1525/elementa.310/.

208 *feed all 327 million Americans:* Shepon, Alon, Gidon Eshel, Elad Noor, and Ron Milo, "The Opportunity Cost of Animal Based Diets Exceeds All Food Losses," *Proceedings of the National Academy of Sciences* 115, no. 15 (March 2018): 3804–3809, https://www.pnas.org/content/115 /15/3804.

208 *"More accurately":* A Well-Fed World, "Scarcity v. Distribution, & the Impact of Animal-Based Foods," 2020, https://awellfedworld.org/scar city-vs-distribution/.

209 *821 million:* Food and Agriculture Organization of the United Nations, "Hunger and Food Insecurity," 2020, http://www.fao.org/hunger/en/.

209 *almost fifteen thousand:* "World Child Hunger Facts—World Hunger Education," World Hunger News, accessed October 3, 2019, https://www .worldhunger.org/world-child-hunger-facts/.

209 *36 percent of the calories:* Emily S. Cassidy, Paul C. West, James S. Gerber, and Jonathan A. Foley, "Redefining Agricultural Yields: From Tonnes to People Nourished per Hectare," *Environmental Research Letters* 8, no. 3 (August 2013), https:// iopscience.iop.org/article/10.1088/1748–9326 /8/3/034015.

209 *"Livestock's Long Shadow":* Food and Agriculture Organization of the United Nations, "Livestock's Long Shadow," 2006, http://www .fao.org/3/a0701e/a0701e00.htm.

We Love

Our

Contributors!

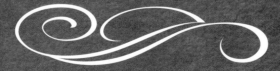

At VegNews, we work with a rockstar team of writers, editors, and photographers from around the globe to deliver the very best experience to our readers. Following are the individuals who contributed to The **VegNews** Guide to Being a Fabulous Vegan, *all to whom we are eternally grateful.* **There would be no book without them!**

The Recipes.

Bacon, Egg & Cheese Breakfast Boat
Recipe by Brian L. Patton
Photography by Veronica Kablan

Baja Cauliflower Tacos with Mango Relish
Recipe by Eddie Garza
Photography by Steven Seighman

BBQ Oyster Mushroom Sliders
Recipe by Jenné Claiborne
Photography by Jenné Claiborne

Beefy Argentinean Empanadas
Recipe by Lauren Kretzer
Photography by Christopher Miller & Kristy Turner

Best Ever Mac & Cheese
Recipe by Allison Rivers Samson
Photography by Hannah Kaminsky

Black-Eyed Pea Croquettes with Creamy Rémoulade Sauce
Recipe by Spork Foods
Photography by Kate Lewis

Boeuf Bourguignon
Recipe by Miyoko Schinner
Photography by Vanessa K. Rees

Candied Blood Orange Cake with Vanilla Bean Buttercream
Recipe by Jackie Sobon
Photography by Jackie Sobon

Cheesy Twice-Baked Potatoes
Recipe by Julie Hasson
Photography by Hannah Kaminsky

Chinese Vegetable Tofu Fried Rice
Recipe by Julie Hasson
Photography by Christopher Miller & Kristy Turner

Chocolate Almond Oat Power Bars
Recipe by Angela Liddon
Photography by Riley Yahr

Chocolate Chile Truffles
Recipe by Fran Costigan
Photography by Kate Lewis

Classic Beefy Burger
Recipe by Joni Marie Newman
Photography by Jackie Sobon

Curried Yellow Lentil Soup
Recipe by Robin Robertson

Deviled Egg Baked Potatoes
Recipe by Julie Hasson
Photography by Christopher Miller & Kristy Turner

Easy Homemade Vegan Milks
Recipes by Sarah McLaughlin

Grilled Bacon Mac & Cheese Sandwiches
Recipe by Jackie Sobon
Photography by Jackie Sobon

Grilled Peach & Tempeh Kebabs
Recipe by Spork Foods
Photography by Jeff & Erin Wysocarski

Heavenly Dark Chocolate Torte
Recipe by Beverly Lynn Bennett
Photography by Hannah Kaminsky

Lavender Sugar Scrub and the Peppermint Body Balm
Recipes by Aurelia d'Andrea

Lemon Blackberry Cupcakes
Recipe by Chloe Coscarelli
Photography by Heather DeVincent

Lemon Pesto Omelet
Recipe by Annie Shannon
Photography by Vanessa K. Rees

Pineapple-Habanero Bean Tacos
Recipe by Stephanie Bogdanich
Photography by Kate Lewis

Middle Eastern Farro Salad with Avocado & Za'atar Feta
Recipe by Julie Morris
Photography by Oliver Barth

Raspberry Almond Butter Oatmeal Bowl
Recipe by Julie Morris
Photography by Oliver Barth

Roasted Cauliflower Steaks with White Wine Cream Sauce
Recipe by Julie Hasson
Photography by Jeff & Erin Wysocarski

Salted Caramel Brownies

Recipe by Jackie Sobon

Photography by Jackie Sobon

Spicy Vegan Chorizo Burrito Bowl

Recipe by Spork Foods

Photography by Christopher Miller & Kristy Turner

Two-Step Biscuits

Recipe by Joni Marie Newman

Photography by Hannah Kaminsky

Vegan Tofu Bánh Mì

Recipe by Robin Robertson

Photography by Hannah Kaminsky

Additional Reporting By

Aurelia d'Andrea

Richard Bowie

Stacy De-Lin

Tanya Flink

Mark Hawthorne

Ellen Kanner

Sarah McLaughlin

David Robinson Simon

Aruka Sanchir

Anna Starostinetskaya

Thank you!

Acknowledgments

Jasmin Singer & VegNews would like to thank . . .

Bringing a

book to life takes dozens of people, and we are so incredibly grateful to those who helped us make this dream a reality.

Thank you to everyone at Foundry Media, including Peter McGuigan, for helping to shape this book in the early days. Huge, gigantic, otherworldly thanks to our incredible (and incredibly unflappable) agent, Claire Harris, for offering so many guideposts on this journey, and for always being so supportive and smart. We are also thankful to Sara DeNobrega, Deirdre Smerillo, Melissa Moorehead, Hayley Burdett, Jessica Felleman, Sarah Lewis, and Yona Levin.

We couldn't have asked for a better editor than Renée Sedliar, who brought tremendous insight, whimsy, and experience to this process. Thanks for believing in this from day one; it's been an honor to work with you. Thanks to the whole team at Hachette Go, including Alison Dalafave, Cisca Schreefel, and designer Tabitha Lahr. Special thanks to Mary Ann Naples, Michelle Aielli, Michael Barrs, and Amanda Kain.

The immensely talented and passionate VegNews team is the reason why this book exists in the first place, and we are so lucky to have them as part of our family. That includes Colleen Holland, Richard Bowie, Anna Starostinetskaya, Sarah McLaughlin, Aruka Sanchir, Aurelia d'Andrea, Joni Marie Newman, Nicole Axworthy, Tanya Flink, Nicholas Holland, Emily Utne, Laurie Johnston, Sutton Long, Laurie Bradley, Carol Treacy, and Lyndsay Orwig. Big thanks, too, to our rockstar writers Ellen Kanner, Mark Hawthorne, and Stacy De-Lin. In addition, we want to give a huge thanks to our incredibly gifted recipe contributors and photographers for this book. We couldn't have done it without you!

In addition, Jasmin Singer would like to thank . . .

There were so many brilliant and generous people who were instrumental in this book coming together. They include Matt Ruscigno, Rachel McCrystal, Maya Gottfried, Andy and Gina Kalish, David Robinson Simon, Joni Marie Newman, Virginia Messina, the woman on the Amtrak train who brought me extra caffeine during my cross-country writing trip, and my best friend and confidante, Erica Nielsen.

Much of the advice you read comes from my own thought process from being a longtime vegan and animal-rights activist. My thoughts were (and remain) heavily influenced by animal law professor and activist Mariann Sullivan, who—amongst many other things—cohosts the Our Hen House podcast each week with me (she also hosts the Animal Law Podcast). We have given countless workshops together over the past many years (I usually let her handle the hard questions), and many of the concepts you just read were the result of me letting Mariann's way of seeing things percolate, and then putting that on paper. Her support in the process of writing this book was vital and deeply appreciated.

While we're on the subject, thank you to the outstanding Our Hen House team, including John Frusciante, Laurie Johnston, Eric Milano, Ben Braman, Elisa Camahort-Page, Rachel Krantz, and—mostly—to our podcast listeners (and darling flock members) who allowed me to yammer on and on each week about writing this. Special thanks to Kathy Head for always supporting and believing in our work. Thanks, too, to the dynamite Kinder Beauty team, including my friends and colleagues Andrew Bernstein, Evanna Lynch, and Daniella Monet.

My genius research assistant Tanya Flink not only gave me an expert take when it came to the health and fitness chapters (having your book assistant be a badass personal trainer is quite the perk), but her many skills in writing, editing, and offering the millennial sign-off were paramount to this project. I'm so beyond grateful, and this book would not be what it is without her impeccable talent.

Thanks to the iconic Milo Runkle for the idea that sparked this book and for making sure I was set up for success. Thanks, too, to Marisa Miller Wolfson, and Amy Scholder. A special thank you to my mom, Roni Omohundro, for always being in my corner—and for reading everything I've ever written in my entire life.

My partner in this project is the incomparable Colleen Holland, VegNews' co-founder and publisher, and my very dear friend. Thanks for the cheerleading texts while I was writing, the endless reasons to raise a glass, and for the beautiful gift of your trust. There is nobody else in the world I could imagine doing this with; you make everything better.

Thanks to my super-supportive wife, Moore Rhys (vegan for twenty-seven years), for letting me bend her ear over and over; for the endless soy lattes (especially when I was on deadline); and for always offering a different perspective. I owe you so much.

And thanks to Lucy Dog, George Dog, and Birdie Dog for making sure I got out every day when all I wanted to do was hole up and write, and to Stella Cat for reminding me how to assert myself when I needed to.

This book is dedicated to Rose, the sweetest and best pitbull I have ever known.

GENERAL INDEX

RECIPE INDEX